Breast Disease

CLINICAL SURGERY INTERNATIONAL

CLINICAL SURGERY INTERNATIONAL

Vol 10   **Breast Disease**

EDITED BY

JOHN F. FORBES

First Assistant, University of Melbourne
Department of Surgery, Royal Melbourne
Hospital, Victoria, Australia

CHURCHILL LIVINGSTONE
EDINBURGH LONDON MELBOURNE AND NEW YORK 1986

CHURCHILL LIVINGSTONE
Medical Division of Longman Group Limited

Distributed in the United States of America by Churchill
Livingstone Inc., 1560 Broadway, New York, N.Y. 10036, and
by associated companies, branches and representatives
throughout the world.

First published 1986

ISBN 0 443 03078 2
ISSN 0203 4422

British Library Cataloguing in Publication Data
Breast disease.—(Clinical surgery international,
    ISSN 0203—4422; v. 10)
    1. Breast—Cancer
    I. Forbes, John F   II. Series
    616.99′449   RC280.B8

Library of Congress Cataloging in Publication Data

Breast disease.

    (Clinical surgery international; vol. 10)
    Includes index.
    1. Breast—Cancer. I. Forbes, John F. (John
Frederick), 1944–   . II. Series: Clinical surgery
international; v. 10.
    RC280.B8B7135   1986   616.99′449   85-17452

Printed at The Bath Press, Avon

Preface

Breast disease has traditionally been treated by surgeons. No other discipline has seen so much relevant new information emerge recently for the understanding of normal function and disease in general and breast cancer in particular. Breast cancer is a 'battlefield' where new and potentially dramatic discoveries in molecular biology are being applied to patient care. Hence, it is not surprising that this volume on breast disease has contributions from experts from a variety of disciplines.

The endocrine control of normal breast tissue and breast cancer is continually promising therapeutic advances. Together with the in vitro studies described by Dr. Whitehead, the endocrinology of normal breast function provides a scientific basis for generating endocrine treatments, although the relevance of the in vitro studies extends way beyond this to control of growth and differentiation, and viral oncogenes. Breast pain is now a well identified clinical problem. Its aetiology and treatment are being unravelled and both depend also on endocrine mechanism as described by Dr. Mansel.

The problem of who will develop breast cancer and by what mechanism, now encompasses discussions of molecular biology and oncogenes (Dr. Dunn), the definition of the risk profile (Dr. Boyd), and the important group of patients with a family history who have a genetically-determined increased risk of developing breast cancer (Dr. King). We can anticipate wider relevance of these areas in the immediate future.

Sound management is dictated by the results of trials. Professor Baum's review serves to remind us of the extent of developments and changes in management that have occurred in the last decade. Although it is accepted that prospective randomised clinical trials provide the best basis for evaluating therapies, it is not always clear what the optimal requirements for such clinical trials in breast cancer are. Dr. Gelber and Dr. Goldhirsch's unique contribution, highlights the importance of a relevant clinical knowledge to the statistician who is going to be involved with breast cancer trials. The data from adjuvant chemotherapy trials and local treatment trials are put into perspective in their appropriate chapters. Management of problems for the patient first presenting, and the patient with locally advanced disease requires sound judgement as well.

This judgement is synthesized in the chapters on practical management and locally advanced disease.

Future management of breast cancer cannot remain the province of the surgeon alone. It has been the aim of this book to indicate the breadth of relevant research and clinical work that is being focused on patients with breast disease and breast cancer. It is hoped that this volume will assist surgeons in particular to gain a broader understanding of management of all patients with breast disease.

Melbourne,   J.F.F.
1986

Contributors

Michael Baum ChM, FRCS
Professor of Surgery, King's College Hospital Medical School, University of London; Honorary Director, CRC Clinical Trials Centre London, UK

N. F. Boyd MB BS FRCP(C)
Clinical Epidemiologist, Ludwig Institute for Cancer Research, Princess Margaret Hospital, Toronto; Associate Professor of Medicine, University of Toronto, Toronto, Canada

Ben W. Davis MD
Assistant Professor of Pathology, Vanderbilt University, Nashville, USA

Ashley R. Dunn PhD
Head, Molecular Biology Group, Ludwig Institute for Cancer Research, Melbourne Tumour Biology Unit, P.O. Royal Melbourne Hospital, Melbourne, Australia

Colin M. Furnival MB ChB PhD FRCS FRACS
Former Associate Professor of Surgery, University of Queensland; Visiting Surgeon, Royal Brisbane Hospital, Brisbane, Australia

Richard D. Gelber PhD
Associate Professor of Biostatistics, Dana-Farber Cancer Institute and Harvard School of Public Health, Boston, USA

Aron Goldhirsch MD
PD, University of Berne; Associate Director for Clinical Activities, Ludwig Institute for Cancer Research, Inselspital, Berne, Switzerland

Mary Claire King PhD
Professor of Epidemiology, School of Public Health, Department of Biomedical and Environmental Health Sciences, University of California, Berkeley, USA

Allan O. Langlands FRCR, FRACR, FRCS (Ed)
Professor of Radiation Oncology, The University of Sydney; Director of
Radiation Oncology, Westmead Hospital, Westmead, New South Wales,
Australia

C. Fred LeMaistre MD
Assistant Professor, Department of Medicine, University of Texas, Health
Science Centre of San Antonio, San Antonio, USA

William L. McGuire MD
Professor of Medicine, Department of Medical Oncology, University of Texas,
Health Science Centre of San Antonio, San Antonio, USA

Robert Mansel MB, BS (Lond), FRCS
Senior Lecturer in Surgery, University of Wales College of Medicine, Cardiff;
Honorary Consultant in General Surgery, South Glamorgan AHA(T), Wales

John S. Simpson MA MB BChir FRCS FRACS
Senior Lecturer, Department of Surgery, Wellington Clinical School of
Medicine, Wellington, New Zealand

R. J. C. Steele MD FRCS (Ed)
Lecturer, University Department of Clinical Surgery, The Royal Infirmary,
Edinburgh, UK

Robert Whitehead MSc, PhD
Head, Cellular Biology Group, Ludwig Institute for Cancer Research,
Melbourne Tumour Biology Unit, P.O. Royal Melbourne Hospital,
Melbourne, Australia

Contents

1 Function of the normal breast: physiology and endocrine control

COLIN M. FURNIVAL

Introduction

In physiological terms the breast is a functional organ which in most women spends the major part of its life between adolescent development and involution, in a resting state. The establishment of normal function (lactation), is determined by the hormonal changes which accompany pregnancy and parturition; once established, lactation may be prolonged for several years by continued suckling. Such prolongation of lactation according to social custom acts as a contraceptive (Howie & McNeilly, 1982), thus establishing a second major role for the breast in the biology of reproduction.

The adult breast has three components which respond to hormone stimulation—stroma, ductal epithelium and myo-epithelial cells. No specific hormonal effects on the vasculature of the breast have been identified. Two classes of hormones primarily influence the state of the breast—oestrogens and progestogens. Hormones which have a specific role in lactation include prolactin, placental lactogen, and oxytocin; other hormones which are necessary for lactation include corticosteroids, insulin and thyroxine.

The morphological basis for hormone effects

Unlike the terminology of breast disease, there is little variation in the nomenclature of the breast structure. The naming of lobules, ducts and lactiferous sinuses is universal and has been clearly defined with reference to pathological changes by Azzopardi (1979). The 'terminal duct–lobular unit' which is the functional unit of the breast refers to the entity of each lobule, consisting of acinar glands, myoepithelial cells and connective tissue together with its adjacent duct (Fig. 1.1). Individual ducts become confluent, like the tributaries of a river, to flow eventually into the dozen or so lactiferous sinuses and the collecting ducts of the nipple.

The ducts and acini are lined by two distinctly different types of cells. The epithelial cells which in the functional state secrete milk, form the luminal

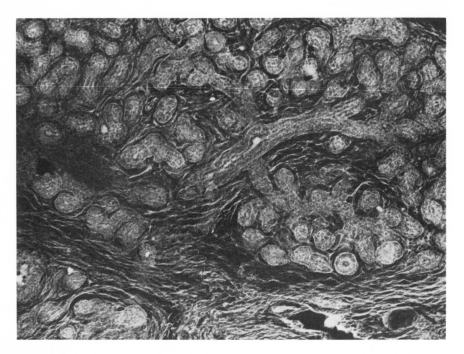

Fig. 1.1 Micro-radiograph showing ductal and acinar pattern in a thick section (50μ) of resting human breast. (Courtesy of Dr J. Pye and Mr R. Davies, Departments of Surgery and Radiology, Welsh National School of Medicine) (× 30).

surface of the acinus; lying peripheral to the epithelial cells are the myo-epithelial cells which are involved in the milk-ejection phenomenon.

The luminal surface of each acinar epithelial cell is convex with numerous microvilli as shown in Figure 1.2 (Hallowes & Peachey, 1980; Halter et al 1981). Ultrastructural studies of these epithelial cells show ribosomes, rough endoplasmic reticulum and in the resting breast, few mitochondria (Ozzello, 1971). Adjacent cell membranes show desmosomes and tight junctions; cell communication is evidenced by gap junctions. The changes which occur in the cytoplasm and its organelles during lactation are described on page 11.

The myo-epithelial cells can be identified by staining for myosin (Gusterson et al, 1982), which shows their relationship to the basement membrane and epithelial cells (Fig. 1.3). Electron micrographs show numerous filaments running parallel to the long axis of the cell (Ozzello, 1971): these are almost certainly the actin and myosin filaments which characterize myo-epithelial cells and blunt projections on the basement membrane side of the cells may form an anchorage during contraction (Ozzello, 1970).

Electron microscopy of the basement membrane shows a monolayer basal lamina together with connective tissue fibres. Proteins contained in the basement membrane include laminin and type IV collagen: studies in the rat show laminin in the cytoplasm of myo-epithelial cells (Warburton et al, 1982), suggesting that the basement membrane proteins may be synthesised by these cells, probably under hormonal control (Liotta et al, 1979).

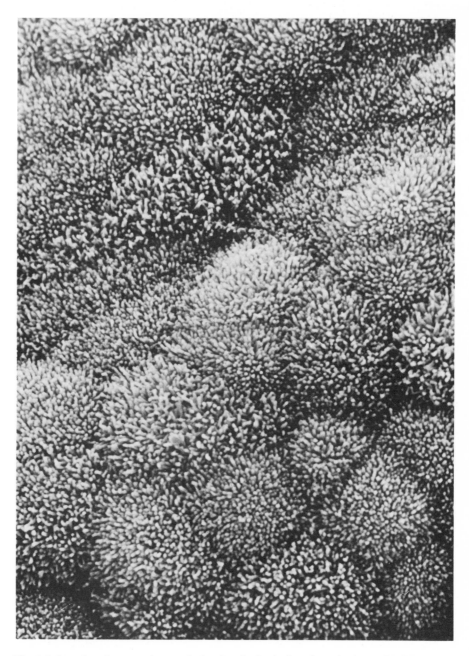

Fig. 1.2 Scanning electron micrograph showing the luminal surface of acinar epithelial cells with micro-villi, in normal breast tissue from a 23 year old woman. (Courtesy of Dr R. C. Hallowes, Imperial Cancer Research Fund, London) (× 3000).

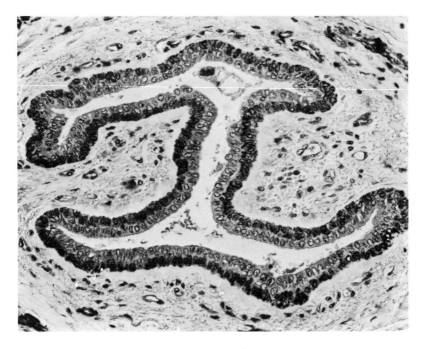

Fig. 1.3 Cross-section of a lactiferous sinus from a resting human breast, stained for myosin by an indirect immuno-cytochemical technique. The darkly staining myo-epithelial cells are peripheral to the lighter epithelial cells. (Courtesy of Dr B. A. Gusterson, Ludwig Institute for Cancer Research, London) (× 250).

The cellular components of the ducts and acini are therefore contained in an 'envelope' consisting of basal lamina, connective tissue fibres and fibroblasts. The network of vascular channels which surrounds the acinus does not cross this layer, so that vital materials must diffuse over a short distance to enter the epithelial cells.

Mechanisms of hormone interaction

The physiological control of breast tissue by circulating hormones is dependent first on the rate of secretion of individual hormones by the parent endocrine gland, second by effective delivery of the hormones to the target organ and finally by an effective interaction between the hormone and the target cell. In the interaction between hormones and their target cells, an important step is the binding of the hormone to specific cytoplasmic or membrane 'receptors'. Whereas hormones readily exhibit binding to non-specific sites (usually proteins) which have a low affinity for the hormone and whose capacity is simply proportional to the hormone concentration, *specific* binding is characterized by high affinity sites with a limited capacity for hormone, often saturated at low concentrations. Early studies of hormone interaction were sometimes confused by non-specific binding. The binding of

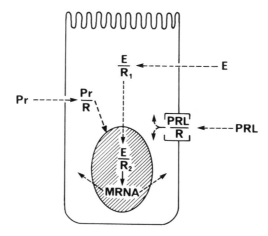

Fig. 1.4 Schematic diagram of hormone interaction in breast epithelial cells. E = oestradiol, Pr = progesterone, PRL = prolactin and R = hormone receptor. Note that the cytoplasmic receptor protein for oestradiol (R_1) has different characteristics than the nuclear receptor protein (R_2). The primary binding site for prolactin appears to be on the cell membrane, not in the cytoplasm.

oestrogen to breast epithelial cells (which has been extensively studied in malignant tumours) provides an example of steroid hormone interaction (Fig. 1.4).

Circulating oestrogen enters the target cell where it binds first to a specific cytoplasmic receptor protein before migrating into the cell nucleus. The effect is to induce gene transcription which is evidenced by the production of messenger RNA within minutes of oestrogen uptake (Means & Hamilton, 1966), followed by an increase in DNA and protein synthesis with mitosis in some cells (Lippman et al, 1976; Edwards, 1981). When human cytoplasmic receptor protein is characterized by sucrose gradient centrifugation, two forms can be detected with sedimentation constants of 8s and 4s (Jensen et al, 1971). The molecular weight of the dominant 8s component is in the region of 200 000 (De Sombre et al, 1971), but after migration to the nucleus, the receptor is identified as having a 5s form suggesting that a transformation of the cytoplasmic receptor has occurred. The significance of this difference is not clear but it allows the definition of both cytoplasmic and nuclear oestrogen receptor proteins whose relevance in malignant breast tissue will be discussed elsewhere.

While the foregoing sequence may be typical of steroid hormones, the receptor sites for polypeptide hormones such as prolactin appear to be located on the plasma membrane rather than in the cytoplasm (Birkinshaw & Falconer, 1972). Although intracellular binding sites have also been described, there seems little doubt that the primary receptor site for prolactin is on the cell membrane (Nagasawa et al 1979).

Binding sites which comply with the definition of 'receptors' (high affinity, low capacity) have now been demonstrated in various preparations of human and animal mammary tissue for oestrogens (Korenman & Dukes, 1970; Gardner & Wittliff, 1973; Hunt & Muldoon, 1977), progesterone (McGuire

& Horwitz, 1978; Wittliff et al, 1978), androgens (Wagner & Jungblut, 1976; Allegra et al, 1979) and prolactin (Costlow & McGuire, 1977; Djiane & Durand, 1977a); specific receptors have also been demonstrated for thyroid hormone, glucocorticoids, insulin and oxytocin.

The action of individual hormones is not easily defined because in life the actions of one hormone may be modified by those of other hormones. For example, the synthesis of progesterone receptor protein in MCF-7 human breast cancer cells is controlled by oestrogens (McGuire & Horwitz, 1978), without which (due to a lack of receptor) progesterone cannot interact with the cell. The observation that progesterone receptor is usually absent from human breast cancers which do not contain oestrogen receptor (Cowan & Lippman, 1982) suggests that this modifying effect of oestrogen may occur generally in breast epithelial cells.

The investigation of hormone interaction in the normal human breast is however limited by the problems of obtaining suitable tissue and by the paucity of epithelial cells in the resting breast (see Fig. 1.6a). The establishment of human ductal epithelial cell cultures provides a useful alternative to breast cancer tissue: conclusions drawn from studies of malignant tissue should not be unreservedly applied to normal epithelial cells because of the phenotypic variation which occurs in cancer cells. At the present time, much of our knowledge of hormone effects is based on animal studies, conclusions from which must also be applied with some caution to the human mammary gland.

Puberty and adolescent development

At about 11 years of age, the primitive breast tissue, nipple and areola begin to show changes which typically progress over the course of 4 years to adult maturity. As in other areas of growth there is substantial variation: the mean age for onset of breast development in English and North American girls is 11.15 years with a standard deviation of 1.10 years (Marshall & Tanner, 1969; Zacharias et al, 1970). Marshall and Tanner describe five stages of visible breast development consisting of progressive enlargement of the breast mound, nipple and areola (stages I–III), transient over-prominence of the nipple and areola (stage IV) and finally maturity (stage V). No further changes occur from this time until pregnancy. This definition of visible stages of development has application in the clinical assessment of endocrine problems, but wide variations obscure a precise definition of normality. Maturity (stage V) is typically reached at 15.3 years but this stage shows the widest variation with a range of 12–19 years.

The visible features of breast development reflect changes in both glandular and connective tissue components of the breast but the principal changes occur in the stroma with the development of adipose tissue amongst the fibrous connective tissue which supports the epithelial element. Dense fibrous tissue around the breast lobules is responsible for the characteristic toughness of young adult breast tissue encountered in surgical procedures.

The epithelial growth which occurs during adolescent development is limited to ductal proliferation and is believed to be stimulated by oestrogens: in the rat, growth hormone and adrenal steroids are also essential and may be necessary in the human female (Lyons, 1958). Lobulo-alveolar development (which is characteristic of pregnancy) does not occur at this time, probably due to a lact of progesterone.

Abnormalities of breast development at this age may reflect hormonal dysfunction particularly if the condition is bilateral. Unilateral absence or hypoplasia of the breast (particularly if associated with absent pectoral muscles) is likely to be due to embryological dysgenesis whereas unilateral hypertrophy may reflect a lack of local control: there appear to be local factors which modify the actions of hormones on developing breast tissue (Knight & Peaker, 1982).

Cyclical changes in the resting breast

The division of the normal menstrual cycle into three phases—menstrual (day 1–5), follicular (day 6–14) and luteal (day 15–30) is based upon characteristic changes in plasma hormones (Fig. 1.5) which also produce cyclical changes in the breast.

Plasma oestradiol is secreted throughout the cycle by the follicular cells of the ovary and by the corpus luteum during the luteal phase; oestrone which has a lower oestrogenic activity than oestradiol is derived from androstenedione, secreted in part by the adrenal gland and shows less variation than oestradiol during the menstrual cycle. The peak plasma oestradiol which occurs at the end of the follicular phase is about four times the basal level at the

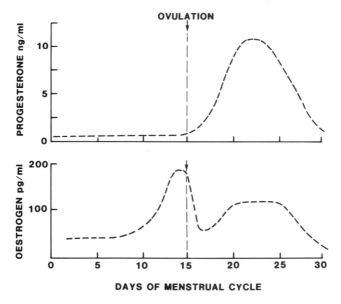

Fig. 1.5 Typical patterns of plasma oestradiol 17-β and progesterone during a normal menstrual cycle (after Mishell et al, 1971).

beginning of the cycle; after the mid-cycle peak, plasma oestradiol is maintained at about twice basal level until menstruation (Mishell et al, 1971).

In contrast to oestrogens, plasma progesterone (and 17α-hydroxyprogesterone) is in low concentration through the follicular phase but rises rapidly after ovulation to a plateau in the mid-luteal phase before declining to basal levels about 5 days before menstruation (Thorneycroft et al, 1971).

The response of the breast to these hormonal fluctuations is shown by changes in volume during each menstrual cycle. Measurements in young women (Milligan et al, 1975) show an increase in volume of 15–30% during the luteal phase of the cycle but there is much individual variation. The decline in volume which begins just before menstruation continues through the follicular phase of the next cycle while oestrogen levels are rising, suggesting that progestogens may be necessary to induce these volume changes. In an oral contraceptive cycle a different pattern is seen, with a sustained increase in volume throughout the hormone phase of the cycle and a rapid decline in volume on cessation of the oestrogen/progesterone combination. These observed changes in volume reflect changes in both the stroma (Ozzello & Speer, 1958), and also the epithelium.

Cyclical changes in the ductal epithelium can be shown by indices of DNA synthesis: measurements of ^{3}H-thymidine uptake in the terminal ductal cells of normal breast tissue show a five-fold increase during the late luteal phase compared with the early follicular phase (Meyer, 1977). The morphological features of these changes include an increase in mitotic rate among lobular epithelial cells towards the end of the cycle with a peak at about day 25 and a cyclical increase in apoptosis (natural cell death) which is maximal about day 28 (Ferguson & Anderson, 1981). Both of these effects occur widely throughout the breasts and oestrogen and progesterone appear to be jointly responsible. The plasma oestrogen which peaks at mid-cycle while plasma progesterone is low evokes no response, but the elevated plasma progesterone during the luteal phase occurs in the presence of twice-basal concentrations of plasma oestradiol.

An important implication of these cyclical changes is that the ductal epithelium is continually renewed. The menstrual cycle shows substantial variation throughout reproductive life and there is some evidence that epithelial cell turnover declines in later reproductive years (Ferguson & Anderson, 1981). This appears to coincide with a rising incidence of breast cancer, which escalates after the menopause when such cyclical changes disappear.

Similar changes in DNA synthesis, peak rates of mitosis and apoptosis are observed during anovulatory cycles induced by the use of oral contraceptives (Meyer, 1977; Anderson et al 1982).

Pregnancy and lactation

Pregnancy

Pregnancy induces a transformation in the breast which prepares it for lactation. Although colostrum may be secreted in the later weeks of pregnancy, true lactation does not begin until after parturition and the sequence of events is conventionally divided into three stages:

1. Mammary growth
2. Lactogenesis (initiation of milk secretion)
3. Lactopoesis (maintenance of lactation)

The escalation of plasma oestrogens which occurs during pregnancy is initiated by the corpus luteum in response to placental HCG, but in the second and third trimesters the placental syncytio-trophoblast appears to be the principal source of oestrogen and progesterone. A high proportion of placental oestrogen is oestrone, a less potent oestrogen than oestradiol (De Hertogh et al, 1975). Nevertheless the increase in oestrogenic effect is as much as 30 times that of the non-pregnant state. Oestrogens are believed to be responsible for ductal development, but a 10-fold increase in plasma progesterone in comparison to luteal phase levels (Klopper & Fuchs, 1977) may be principally responsible for acinar development; the division of labour between these hormones is again difficult to define.

The earliest changes of pregnancy are an increase in breast size which may be the first confirmation of conception: this effect is probably oestrogenic. The rise in plasma oestradiol begins with conception and is three or four times luteal phase values by 20 days, at which time progesterone is still at normal luteal phase levels or even lower (Klopper & Fuchs, 1977). As pregnancy continues, acinar development is established and by the time of parturition the breast shows the typical morphology of lactation (Fig. 1.6b).

In addition to oestrogens and progestogens, the polypeptide hormones prolactin (from the anterior pituitary) and placental lactogen are involved in the breast development of pregnancy. The remarkable structural similarity between prolactin and placental lactogen suggests a similar action in the target organ and a common genetic programme in the pituitary and placental secretory cells. The molecular similarity of both of these hormones to growth hormone (which is essential for mammary development in some animals) suggests that all may have a common action in acinar development.

In rats and mice, acinar development requires prolactin together with the hormones necessary for ductal development, again suggesting a complex integration of hormone actions. In some species prolactin appears to be the dominant hormone, without which little epithelial growth occurs (Stoudemire et al, 1975).

In the human female, prolactin rises 20–30 times during pregnancy (Sadovsky et al, 1977) and placental lactogen which begins to appear in plasma during the first trimester shows a progressive rise up to the time of parturition (Fluckiger, et al, 1982). It would seem reasonable to suggest that teleologically, placental lactogen is an essential factor in the preparation of the human breast for lactation but there is some evidence that lactation can be induced by prolactin in the presence of oestrogen (Tyson et al, 1976). Cases have also been recorded of otherwise normal pregnancies in which placental lactogen is apparently absent (Nielsen, et al, 1979). A common receptor site for prolactin and placental lactogen may well explain these observations but it appears that at

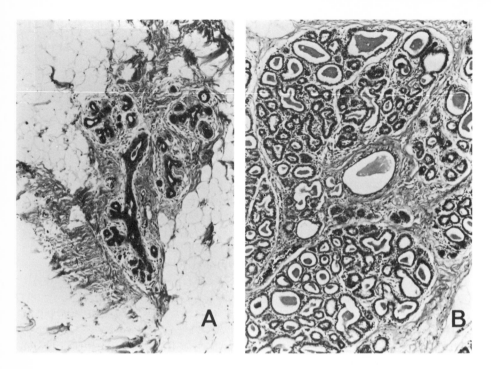

Fig. 1.6 Sections of human adult breast A: ductal pattern with surrounding adipose tissue in a 'resting' breast; B: acinar development in late pregnancy, before lactation (H & E × 15).

least in normal circumstances human placental lactogen has an important role in the preparation of the breast for lactation.

Growth hormone in the human shows little change during pregnancy and is not essential for mammary development.

The changes of pregnancy are accompanied by a substantial increase in blood flow through the breast (Davis et al, 1979), evidenced clinically by increased prominence of the subcutaneous veins. In addition to enlargement and increased vascularity a progressive pigmentation of the areola appears during pregnancy, due to an apparently localized stimulation of melanocytes in this region. Whether these melanocytes respond differently to hormones or benefit from the local delivery of hormones as a result of increased blood flow is not known but the stimulus appears to be oestrogenic: it can be reproduced by therapeutic oestrogens and was often seen when these were used in the treatment of advanced breast cancer.

Lactation

A detailed account of the physiology of lactation is beyond the scope of this chapter (see reviews by Peaker, 1977 and Cowie et al, 1980). In brief, the mammary development of pregnancy is followed by a transitional phase of lactogenesis lasting 4–5 days during which copious milk secretion of up to

400 ml/day is established. The term lactopoesis is used to describe the maintenance of milk secretion.

The initiation of milk secretion after parturition coincides with major changes in plasma hormones, including a reduction in oestrogens and progesterone and an increase in plasma prolactin and corticosteroids (Kulski et al, 1977). The difficulty of ascribing such changes to specific hormones again relates to the interaction of individual hormones: although animal studies suggest that the inhibition of lactation prior to parturition is due to a high plasma progesterone (Djiane & Durand, 1977b), oestrogens have been implicated in the human and may act directly on acinar cells, possibly by inhibiting prolactin receptor synthesis (Bruce & Ramirez, 1970). It is, however, clear that the suppression of prolactin secretion by bromocriptine inhibits lactation (Nilsen et al 1976), and that the return of plasma oestrogen and progesterone to non-pregnant levels is completed before maximal milk secretion occurs (Fluckiger et al, 1982).

Milk has a higher concentration of carbohydrate and a lower concentration of protein than colostrum. The major components, protein, carbohydrate and fatty acids are secreted by the acinar epithelial cells under hormonal control. The milk proteins, casein and lactalbumin are synthesised from plasma amino acids in the ribosomes and the genetic transcription of relevant DNA codes is probably initiated by prolactin (Mepham, 1977). Animal studies suggest that insulin which is essential for this process may control the passage of amino acids from extracellular fluid into the epithelial cells (Anderson & Rillema, 1976) and changes in the rough endoplasmic reticulum have been observed in animal culture following the addition of insulin to the culture medium (Cowie et al, 1980).

After synthesis, proteins are temporarily located in the Golgi apparatus where casein micelles form before their transport to the luminal membrane and release into the acinus. Lactalbumin performs its function in the Golgi apparatus by combining with galactosyl transferase to synthesise lactose from carbohydrate precursors. Lactose, the principle carbohydrate of milk, is subsequently released into the lumen of the gland. Little is known about hormonal control of lactose secretion which may be limited principally by the availability of glucose in the cytoplasm (Jones, 1977).

Synthesis of the fatty acid (triglyceride) component of milk by the epithelial cells appears to be dependent upon insulin, cortisol and prolactin: in small animals the exposure of pregnant mammary tissue to this combination results in a 30- to 40-fold increase in fatty acid synthesis within 24 hours (Speake et al, 1976). Synthesis ceases immediately when these hormones are withdrawn.

The maintenance of milk secretion, dependent upon prolactin, is ensured by repeated suckling which induces the release of prolactin from the anterior pituitary (Hwang et al, 1971; Noel et al, 1974). The absence or withdrawal of this stimulus inhibits lactation in women who do not wish to breast feed.

In addition to the nutritional components, human milk contains a substantial number of epithelial cells and macrophages. It has been known since the last century that immunity can be transferred in the milk and in humans, whose infants obtain IgG via the placenta, the principal immunoglobulin is IgA which is present in slightly higher concentration in colostrum than in milk. This IgA is produced by plasma cells within the mammary gland and its principal function may be to protect the infant against gastrointestinal infection, particularly from *E. coli* (Rogers & Synge, 1978). The plasma cells, which are IgA-secreting B-lymphocytes, originate in the lymphoid tissue of the gut and their localization to the breast in large numbers during lactation appears to be directed by the hormonal changes of pregnancy (McClelland, 1982).

No account of hormonal mechanisms in lactation would be complete without brief reference to the milk ejection phenomenon. The suggestion that the reflex release of milk in response to suckling might be mediated by a hormone was first made by Ely and Peterson in 1941 and the existence of a neuro-endocrine reflex was established beyond doubt in the early 1950's. Afferent impulses from sensory receptors in the nipple provoke the release of oxytocin from the posterior pituitary gland (Drewett et al, 1982): the oxytocin induces rhythmic contractions of the myo-epithelial cells around the ducts and acini, resulting in a rise in pressure which forces milk into the lactiferous sinuses (Cobo et al, 1967). The simultaneous effect in both breasts may produce spurts of milk from the nipple which is not being suckled, an observation immortalized in Greek mythology as the origin of the Galaxy or Milky Way (Fig. 1.7). A detailed account of the afferent component, mechanisms of hormone release and effect has recently been given by Lincoln and Paisley (1982).

The stimulus of suckling therefore has a dual hormonal effect: release of prolactin from the anterior pituitary ensures the continued secretion of milk and release of oxytocin from the posterior pituitary ensures its delivery to the infant.

Involution

The final chapter in the hormonal response of breast tissue is the involution which occurs in two circumstances, a) following the cessation of lactation and b) after the menopause.

When breast feeding is discontinued there is an abrupt reduction in the volume of milk in response to the withdrawal of regular prolactin stimulation. Examination of residual breast secretions shows that lactose concentration declines over a 2–3 week period while casein and lactalbumin are replaced by other proteins including immunoglobulins (Hartmann & Kulski, 1978). Dissolution of the acinar development occurs: necrotic cells and their debris are taken up by numerous macrophages. The earliest changes shown by electron microscopy include fragmentation of fat droplets and the appearance of vacuoles, possibly due to protein digestion, in the epithelial cells (Richards & Benson, 1971). These changes are accompanied in the human female by a gradual reduction in breast size and vascularity together with a return of the nipple and areola to the non-pregnant state.

In the older woman, progressive loss of lobules and ductal structures follows oestrogen reduction at the menopause and is accompanied by replacement of dense connective tissue by adipose tissue (Azzopardi, 1979). The post-meno-

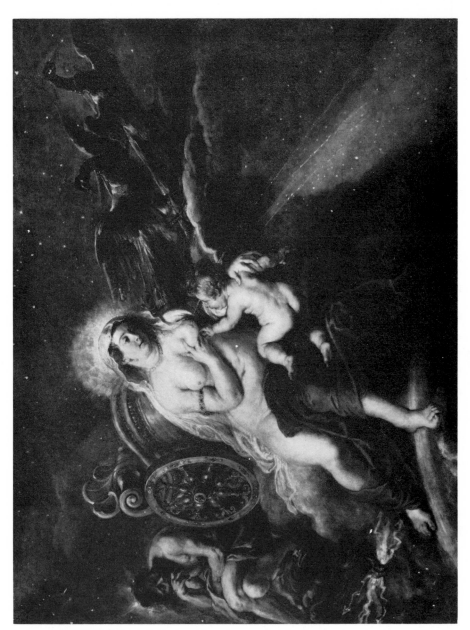

Fig. 1.7 Rubens: 'The Milky Way', depicting the origin of the Galaxy, in Greek legend. (Courtesy of Museo Nacional del Prado, Madrid).

pausal breast thus contains a high proportion of fatty tissue in comparison to the pre-menopausal breast, facilitating the diagnosis of malignant neoplasms by mammography in this age group.

Hormones and benign breast disease

In the absence of any obvious alternative aetiology, many benign breast disorders have been ascribed to disturbed hormone interaction. However, with the exception of galactorrhoea, it has proved difficult to define the hormonal imbalances which may be responsible for benign disease. The difficulties are compounded by the fact that some disorders, which are evidently hormone-related (such as fibrocystic disease), may present as localized lesions: hormone disturbances would be expected to produce a diffuse, general effect on breast tissue.

Little experimental evidence is available to clarify these issues and the lack of a suitable animal model for the study of benign breast pathology is a major impediment to our understanding of these conditions. It is however of interest that when dimethylbenzanthracene is used to induce mammary cancers in Sprague-Dawley rats, nodular hyperplastic changes occur in a proportion of animals, before malignant change appears (Carter, 1984).

When plasma hormones are measured in women with benign disease, most women show only minor variations in hormone levels when compared with normal controls: however, it is possible that small changes in individual hormone concentrations disturb hormone ratios to produce an exaggerated effect upon a highly sensitive target organ. Such a mechanism is supported by the action of oral contraceptive hormones which produce minimal changes in plasma concentrations, but may induce or relieve some types of benign breast disease. The *availability* of plasma hormones may also be a critical factor and abnormalities of oestrogen binding to plasma globulins may influence the oestrogenic effect even when total plasma oestrogen remains normal (Moore et al, 1982).

Mastalgia

Women who suffer cyclical mastalgia frequently show a slight elevation of serum prolactin (Cole et al, 1977). Although values are often within the normal range, cyclical mastalgia is associated with higher mean serum prolactin concentrations than those found in asymptomatic women; serum oestradiol in such women is the same as in normal controls (Watt-Boolsen et al, 1981). The elevation of prolactin is seen during both phases of the menstrual cycle. Paradoxically women with true hyperprolactinaemia resulting in galactorrhoea rarely suffer from mastalgia.

The symptoms of mastalgia can be relieved by inhibiting prolactin secretion with the dopamine agonist bromocriptine (Mansel et al, 1978; Durning & Sellwood, 1982), but can also be relieved by the anti-gonadotrophic effect of danazol (Asch & Greenblatt, 1977; Mansell et al, 1982) and by tamoxifen, presumably acting as an anti-oestrogen (Shaaban, Morad & Hassan, 1980).

Our own observations confirm that tamoxifen is an effective agent for the control of non-cyclical mastalgia, suggesting that oestrogen interaction with the target organ is at least one component in the pathogenesis of painful breast disease.

Fibrocystic disease

Fibrocystic disease has been historically attributed to oestrogen excess and biopsy material contains oestrogen receptor protein, though usually in low concentration (Feherty et al, 1971; Hawkins et al, 1975). However, measurable elevations of plasma oestrogens in women with various forms of fibrocystic disease are less consistent than low plasma progesterone levels during the luteal phase (Sitruk-Ware et al, 1979): such women show a highly significant difference in plasma progesterone/oestradiol ratio in comparison to normal women, again suggesting a complex interaction of hormones on sensitive breast tissue. The low progesterone may be attributed to deficient corpus luteum function and elevation of plasma LH, compatible with defective progesterone secretion, has been observed in women with fibrocystic disease (Golinger et al, 1978). Serum prolactin appears to be normal in this condition.

The transient nature of fibrocystic disease presenting as a breast lump in young women (Furnival et al, 1983) is not incompatible with a hormonal basis but the localized lesion again suggests that other aetiological factors may initiate the pathological change.

The concentration of hormones in breast cyst fluid has been studied in an attempt to elucidate hormonal mechanisms. Steroid hormone metabolites and prolactin have been found in higher concentration in cyst fluid than plasma (Bradlow et al, 1979; Raju et al, 1981), but the implications (if any) for pathogenesis are uncertain. It appears that there are two populations of breast cysts characterized by the lining epithelium (Dixon et al, 1983): cysts lined by secretory apocrine epithelium contain a higher concentration of the adrenal androgen DHA-sulphate than cysts which are lined by flattened epithelium. In women with multiple cysts, one or other type predominates, suggesting an underlying hormonal mechanism.

Fibro-adenoma is typical of the localized benign disease which cannot be easily attributed to hormonal dysfunction. Most fibro-adenomas contain measurable oestrogen receptor protein (Martin et al, 1978) and appear to be sensitive to plasma oestrogens; evidence of such an effect is sometimes seen during pregnancy, but women with fibro-adenomas who use oral contraceptive hormones do not show excessive epithelial proliferation (Fechner, 1970). Multiple fibroadenomas are no more common in women using oral contraceptives than in those who do not and indeed oral contraceptive hormones may give slight protection against benign disease (Vessey et al, 1972).

In general, the histological features of fibrocystic disease among women who take oestrogens are similar to those in women who are not exposed to exogenous hormones (Fechner, 1972).

Mammary duct ectasia

Mammary duct ectasia, unlike fibrocystic disease, appears to be a primary inflammatory condition with secondary ductal changes (Azzopardi, 1979): there does not appear to be an underlying hormonal basis (Dixon et al, 1983).

Galactorrhoea

As a final example of the role of hormones in the pathogenesis of breast disease, galactorrhoea appears to be directly related to prolactin secretion.

Although measurements of plasma prolactin may be normal in as many as 30% of women with galactorrhoea, the remainder show hyperprolactinaemia of varying degrees: the highest levels are found in women with pituitary tumours who comprise about 20% of all patients with galactorrhoea (Tolis et al, 1974; Kleinberg et al, 1977). Other causes of excessive prolactin secretion include the adverse effects of drugs such as chlorpromazine, metoclopramide and domperidone: each of these agents is a dopamine antagonist and administration produces elevation of plasma prolactin (Brouwers et al, 1980). The anti-emetic domperidone is associated with a high incidence of galactorrhoea (Cann et al, 1983) which may appear within 48 hours of administration (Maddern, 1983). Methyldopa can also occasionally induce galactorrhoea, presumably by inhibiting dopamine synthesis (Tolis et al, 1974), and all of these agents can cause gynaecomastia in the male.

Galactorrhoea is controlled in a high proportion of cases by the prolactin inhibitor bromocriptine (Lutterbeck et al, 1971; Kleinberg et al, 1977).

REFERENCES

Allegra J C, Lippman M E, Thomson E B et al 1979 Distribution, frequency and quantitative analysis of estrogen, progesterone, androgen and glucocorticoid receptors in human breast cancer. Journal of Cancer Research 39: 1447–1454
Anderson T J, Ferguson D J P, Raab G M 1982 Cell turnover in the resting human breast: influence of parity, contraceptive pill, age and laterality. British Journal of Cancer 46: 376–382
Anderson L D, Rillema J A 1976 Effects of hormones on protein and amino acid metabolism in mammary gland explants of mice. Biochemical Journal 158: 355–359
Asch R H, Greenblatt R B 1977 The use of an impeded androgen–danazol, in the management of benign breast disorders. American Journal of Obstetrics and Gynecology 127: 130–134
Azzopardi J G 1979 Problems in breast pathology. Saunders, London
Birkinshaw M, Falconer I R 1972 The localisation of prolactin labelled with radioactive iodine in rabbit mammary tissue. Journal of Endocrinology 55: 323–334
Bradlow H L, Schwartz M K, Fleischer M et al 1979 Accumulation of hormones in breast cyst fluid. Journal of Clinical Endocrinology and Metabolism 49: 778–782
Brouwers J R B J, Assies J, Wiersinga W M, Huizing G, Tytgat G N 1980 Plasma prolactin levels after acute and sub-chronic oral administration of domperidone and metoclopramide. Clinical Endocrinology 12: 435–440
Bruce J O, Ramirez V D 1970 Site of action of the inhibitory effect of estrogen upon lactation. Neuroendocrinology 6: 19–29
Cann P A, Read N W, Holdsworth C D 1983 Galactorrhoea as a side effect of domperidone. British Medical Journal 286: 1395–1396
Carter J 1984 Personal communication
Cobo E, de Bernal M M, Gaitan E, Quintero C A 1967 Neurohypophyseal hormone release in the human II: Experimental study during lactation. Journal of Obstetrics and Gynecology 97: 519–529
Cole E N, Sellwood R A, England P C, Griffiths K 1977 Serum prolactin concentrations in

benign breast disease throughout the menstrual cycle. European Journal of Cancer 13: 597–603

Costlow M E, McGuire W L 1977 Autoradiographic localisation of the binding of ^{125}I-labelled prolactin to rat tissues in vitro. Journal of Endocrinology 75: 221–226

Cowan K, Lippman M 1982 Steroid receptors in breast cancer. Archives of Internal Medicine 142: 363–366

Cowie A T, Forsyth I A, Hart I C 1980 Hormonal control of lactation. Monographs on endocrinology 15. Springer-Verlag, Berlin

Davis A J, Fleet I R, Goode J A, Hammon M H, Walker F, Peaker M 1979 Changes in mammary function at the onset of lactation in the goat: correlation with hormonal changes. Journal of Physiology 288: 33–44

De Hertogh R, Thomas K, Bietlo Y, Vanderheyden I, Ferin J 1975 Plasma levels of unconjugated estrone, estradiol and estriol and of HCS throughout pregnancy in normal women. Journal of Clinical Endocrinology and Metabolism 40: 93–101

De Sombre E R, Chabaud G A, Puca G A, Jensen E V 1971 Purification and properties of an estrogen-binding protein from calf uterus. Journal of Steroid Biochemistry 2: 95–103

Dixon J M, Anderson T J, Lumsden A B, Elton R A, Roberts M M, Forrest A P M 1983 Mammary duct ectasia. British Journal of Surgery 70: 601–603

Dixon J M, Miller W R, Scott W N, Forrest A P M 1983 The morphological basis of human breast cyst populations. British Journal of Surgery 70: 604–606

Djiane J, Durand P 1977a Evolution of prolactin receptors in rabbit mammary gland during pregnancy and lactation. Endocrinology 100: 1348–1356

Djiane J, Durand P 1977b Prolactin-progesterone antagonism in self regulation of prolactin receptors in the mammary gland. Nature 266: 641–643

Drewett R F, Bowen-Jones A, Dogterom J 1982 Oxytocin levels during breast feeding in established lactation. Hormones and Behaviour 16: 245–248

Durning P, Sellwood R A 1982 Bromocriptine in severe cyclical breast pain. British Journal of Surgery 69: 248–249

Edwards D P, Adams D J, McGuire W L 1981 Specific protein synthesis regulated by estrogen in human breast cancer. Journal of Steroid Biochemistry 15: 247–259

Fechner R E 1970 Fibro-adenomas in patients receiving oral contraceptives. A clinical and pathological study. American Journal of Clinical Pathology 53: 857–864

Fechner R E 1972 Benign breast disease in women on estrogen therapy: a pathologic study. Cancer 29: 273–279

Feherty P, Farrer-Brown G, Kellie A E 1971 Oestradiol receptors in carcinoma and benign disease of the breast: an in vitro assay. British Journal of Cancer 25: 697–710

Ferguson D J P, Anderson T J 1981 Morphological evaluation of cell turnover in relation to the menstrual cycle in the resting human breast. British Journal of Cancer 44: 177–181

Fluckiger E, del Pozo E, von Werder K 1982 Prolactin. Monographs on Endocrinology 23 Springer-Verlag, Berlin. p 67

Furnival C M, Irwin J R M, Gray G 1983 Breast lumps in young women: when is biopsy indicated? Medical Journal of Australia 2: 167–169

Gardner D G, Wittliff J L 1973 Specific estrogen receptors in the lactating mammary gland of the rat. Biochemistry 12: 3090–3096

Golinger R C, Krebs J, Fisher E R, Danowski T S 1978 Hormones and the pathophysiology of fibrocystic mastopathy: elevated luteinizing hormone levels. Surgery 84: 212–215

Gusterson B A, Warburton M J, Mitchell D, Ellison M, Neville A M, Rudland P S 1982 Distribution of myo-epithelial cells and basement membrane proteins in the normal breast and in benign and malignant breast diseases. Cancer Research 42: 4763–4770

Hallowes R C, Peachey L A 1980 The mammary gland and human breast. In: Hodges G M, Hallowes R C (eds) Biomedical Research Applications of Scanning Electron Microscopy 2, p 167

Halter S A, Holt D H, Page D L 1981 Hyperplastic lesions of the human breast: scanning electron microscopy and a review of current knowledge. Scanning Electron Microscopy 3: 11–22

Hartmann P E, Kulski J K 1978 Changes in the composition of the mammary secretion of women after abrupt termination of breast feeding. Journal of Physiology 275: 1–11

Hawkins R A, Hill A, Freedman B 1975 A simple method for the determination of oestrogen receptor concentrations in breast tumours and other tissues. Clinical Chemistry Acta 64: 203–210

Howie P W, McNeilly A S 1982 Effect of breast feeding patterns on human birth intervals. Journal of Reproduction and Fertility 65: 545–557

Hunt M E, Muldoon T G 1977 Factors controlling oestrogen receptor levels in normal mouse mammary tissue. Journal of Steroid Biochemistry 8: 181–186

Hwang P, Guyda H, Friesen H 1971 A radioimmunoassay for human prolactin. Proceedings of the National Academy of Sciences (New York) 68: 1902–1906

Jensen E V, Block G E, Smith S, Kyser K, De Sombre E R 1971 Estrogen receptors and breast cancer response to adrenalectomy. National Cancer Institute Monographs 34: 55–70

Jones E A 1977 Synthesis and secretion of milk sugars. In: Peaker M (ed) Comparative Aspects of Lactation (Zoological Society of London Symposium No 41), Academic Press, London. p 77

Kleinberg D L, Noel G L, Frantz A G 1977 Galactorrhoea: A study of 235 cases including 48 with pituitary tumours. New England Journal of Medicine 296: 589–600

Klopper A, Fuchs F 1977 Progestagens. In: Fuchs F, Klopper A (eds) Endocrinology of Pregnancy, 2nd edn. Harper and Row, London. p 99

Knight C H, Peaker M 1982 Development of the mammary gland. Journal of Reproduction and Fertility 65: 521–536

Korenman S G, Dukes B A 1970 Specific oestrogen binding by the cytoplasm of human breast carcinoma. Journal of Clinical Endocrinology and Metabolism 30: 639–645

Kulski J K, Smith M, Hartmann P E 1977 Perinatal concentrations of progesterone, lactose and α-lactalbumin in the mammary secretion of women. Journal of Endocrinology 74: 509–510

Lincoln D W, Paisley A C 1982 Neuroendocrine control of milk ejection. Journal of Reproduction and Fertility 65: 571–586

Liotta L A, Wicha M S, Foidart J M, Rennard S I, Garbisa S, Kidwell W R 1979 Hormonal requirements for basement membrane collagen deposition by cultured rat mammary epithelium. Laboratory Investigation 41: 511–518

Lippman M, Bolan G, Huff K 1976 The effects of estrogens and anti-estrogens on hormone responsive human breast cancer in long term tissue culture. Cancer Research 36: 4595–4601

Lutterbeck P M, Pryor J S, Varga L, Wenner R 1971 Treatment of non-puerperal galactorrhoea with an ergot alkaloid. British Medical Journal 3: 228–229

Lyons W R 1958 Hormonal synergism in mammary growth. Proceedings of the Royal Society (Biology) 149: 303–325

Maddern G J 1983 Galactorrhoea due to domperidone. Medical Journal of Australia 2: 539–540

Mansel R E, Preece P E, Hughes L E 1978 A double-blind trial of the prolactin inhibitor bromocriptine in painful benign breast disease. British Journal of Surgery 65: 724–727

Mansel R E, Wisbey J R, Hughes L E 1982 Controlled trial of the anti-gonadotrophin danazol in painful nodular breast disease. Lancet 1: 928–930

Marshall W A, Tanner J M 1969 Variations in pattern of pubertal changes in girls. Archives of Diseases of Childhood 44: 291–303

Martin P M, Kuttenn F, Serment H, Mauvais-Jarvis P 1978 Studies on clinical hormonal and pathological correlations in breast fibro-adenomas. Journal of Steroid Biochemistry 9: 1251–1255

McClelland D B L 1982 Antibodies in milk. Journal of Reproduction and Fertility 65: 537–543

McGuire W L, Horwitz K B 1978 Progesterone receptors in breast cancer. In: McGuire W L (ed) Progress in Cancer Research and Therapy. 10: Hormones, Receptors and Breast Cancer. Raven Press, New York p 31

Means A R, Hamilton T H 1966 Early estrogen action: concomitant stimulations within two minutes of nuclear RNA synthesis and uptake of RNA precursor by the uterus. Proceedings of the National Academy of Sciences (New York) 56: 1594–1598

Mepham T B 1977 Synthesis and secretion of milk proteins. In: Peaker M (ed) Comparative Aspects of Lactation (Zoological Society of London Symposium No 41), Academic Press, London. p 57

Meyer J S 1977 Cell proliferation in normal human breast ducts, fibro-adenomas and other ductal hyperplasias measured by nuclear labelling with tritiated thymidine. Human Pathology 8: 67–81

Milligan D, Drife, J O, Short R V 1975 Change in breast volume during normal menstrual cycle and after oral contraceptives. British Medical Journal 4: 494–496

Mishell D R, Nakamura R M, Crosignani P G et al 1971 Serum gonadotropin and steroid patterns during the normal menstrual cycle. American Journal of Obstetrics and Gynecology 111: 60–65

Moore J W, Clark G M G, Bulbrook R D et al 1982 Serum concentrations of total and non-protein bound oestradiol in patients with breast cancer and in normal controls. International Journal of Cancer 29: 17–21

Nagasawa H, Sakai S, Banerjee M R 1979 Prolactin receptors. Life Science 24: 193–208

Nielsen P V, Pedersen H, Kampmann E M 1979 Absence of human placental lactogen in an otherwise uneventful pregnancy. American Journal of Obstetrics and Gynecology 135: 322–326

Nilsen P A, Meling A-B, Abildgaard U 1976 Study of the suppression of lactation and the influence on blood clotting with bromocriptine: a double-blind comparison with diethylstilboestrol. Acta obstetrics and Gynaecology Scandavica 55: 39–44

Noel G L, Suh H K, Frantz A G 1974 Prolactin release during nursing and breast stimulation in post-partum and non-post-partum subjects. Journal of Clinical Endocrinology and Metabolism 38: 413–423

Ozzello L 1971 Epithelial-stromal junction of normal and dysplastic mammary glands. Cancer 25: 586–600

Ozzello L 1970 Ultrastructure of the human mammary gland. In: Sommers S C (ed) Pathology Annual 6. Butterworths, London. p 1

Ozzello L, Speer F D 1958 The mucopolysaccharides in the normal and diseased breast. American Journal of Pathology 34: 993–1005

Peaker M 1977 Comparative aspects of lactation (Zoological Society of London Symposium No 41). Academic Press, London

Raju U, Noumoff J, Levitz M, Bradlow H L, Breed C N 1981 On the occurrence and transport of oestriol-3-sulfate in human breast cyst fluid. Journal of Clinical Endocrinology and Metabolism 53: 847–851

Richards R C, Benson G K 1971 Ultrastructural changes accompanying involution of the mammary gland in the albino rat. Journal of Endocrinology 51: 127–135

Rogers H J, Synge C 1978 Bacteriostatic effect of human milk on Escherichia coli: the role of IgA. Immunology 34: 19–28

Sadovsky E, Weinstein D, Ben-David M, Polishuk W Z 1977 Serum prolactin in normal and pathologic pregnancy. Obstetrics and Gynaecology 50: 559–561

Shaaban M M, Morad F, Hassan A R 1980 Treatment of fibrocystic mastopathy by an anti-oestrogen, tamoxifen. International Journal of Gynaecology and Obstetrics 18: 348–350

Sitruk-Ware R, Sterkers N, Mauvais-Jarvis P 1979 Benign breast disease I: hormonal investigation. Obstetrics and Gynaecology 53: 457–460

Speake B K, Dils R, Mayer R J 1976 Effect of hormones on lipogenesis in mammary explants taken from rabbits at different stages of pregnancy and lactation. Biochemical Society Transactions 4: 238–240

Stoudemire G A, Stumpf W E, Sar M 1975 Synergism between prolactin and ovarian hormones on DNA synthesis in rat mammary gland. Proceedings of the Society for Experimental Biology and Medicine 149: 189–192

Thorneycroft I H, Mishell D R, Stone S C, Kharma K M, Nakamura R M 1971 The relation of serum 17-hydroxyprogesterone and oestradiol-17β levels during the human menstrual cycle. American Journal of Obstetrics and Gynecology 111: 947–951

Tolis G, Somma M, Van Campenhout J, Friesen H 1974 Prolactin secretion in 65 patients with galactorrhoea. American Journal of Obstetrics and Gynecology 118: 91–101

Tyson J E, Freedman R S, Perez A, Zacur H A, Zanartu J 1976 Significance of the secretion of human prolactin and gonadotrophin for puerperal lactational infertility. CIBA Foundation Symposium 45: 49–64

Vessey M P, Doll R, Sutton P M 1972 Oral contraceptives and breast neoplasia: a retrospective study. British Medical Journal 3: 719–724

Wagner R K, Jungblut P W 1976 Oestradiol and dihydrotestosterone receptors in normal and neoplastic human mammary tissue. Acta Endocrinologica 82: 105–120

Warburton M J, Mitchell D, Ormerod E J, Rudland P 1982 Distribution of myo-epithelial cells and basement membrane proteins in the resting, pregnant, lactating and involuting rat mammary gland. Journal of Histochemistry and Cytochemistry 30: 667–676

Watt-Boolsen S, Andersen A N, Blichert-Toft M 1981 Serum prolactin and oestradiol levels in women with cyclical mastalgia. Hormone and Metabolism Research 13: 700–702

Wittliff J L, Lewko W M, Park D C et al 1978 Steroid binding proteins of mammary tissues and their clinical significance in breast cancer. In: McGuire W L (ed) Progress in Cancer Research and Therapy 10: Hormones, Receptors and Breast Cancer, Raven Press, New York p 325

Zacharias L, Wurtman R J, Schatzuff M 1970 Sexual maturation in contemporary American girls. American Journal of Obstetrics and Gynecology 108: 833–846

2 The histogenesis of breast tissue and the growth of normal, benign and malignant breast tissue in vitro

R. H. WHITEHEAD

The culture of breast cells in vitro is rendered more difficult by the hormonal dependence of this tissue. Although histologically the breast is relatively simple with only two main epithelial cell types (secretory epithelial and myoepithelial) the picture is rendered more complex by the multiple changes that occur during a lifetime: initial development, puberty, pregnancy, lactation, weaning, menopause and post-menopausal atrophy. No in vitro model can hope to mimic all of these conditions and very little has been done to try to duplicate the hormonal mileau relevant to these different in vivo states.

Embryology

The breast region first becomes recognisable in the developing embryo with the appearance of a 2–4 cell-layered ectodermal mammary streak at 5 weeks. At about the seventh week of intrauterine growth the mammary ridge is formed in the thoracic region and the remainder of the mammary streak regresses. The ectodermal tissue then begins to invaginate the underlying mesenchymal tissue and begins to grow in three dimensions. The descending tips of ectoderm branch until between 15–25 epithelial strips are formed and these later canalise and give rise to the mammary ducts. The formation of glandular lumina begins at the periphery of the epithelial strips and proceeds centrally. Simultaneously with the epithelial development, increased vascularisation and formation of connective tissue and fat are observed. After birth the breast tissue regresses somewhat and remains essentially quiescent until puberty.

During childhood the structure of the ductal and alveolar tissue is simple with a two cell-layered lining epithelium being surrounded by myoepithelial cells. Under the influences of sterioids, especially oestrogen, the mammary glandular epithelium proliferates and ductal and alveolar epithelium can be readily distinguished with the latter taking on all the ultrastructural appearances of secretory cells. The myoepithelial cells surrounding the alveoli and

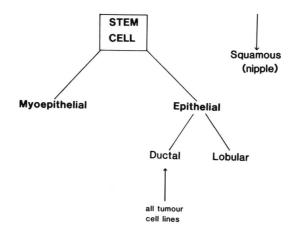

Fig. 2.1 Probable differentiation pathway of the epithelial cells of the breast. The similarity of breast carcinoma cell lines to cells in this differentiation lineage is indicated (see text).

ducts also increase in number under similar stimuli. There is some debate as to whether epithelial and myoepithelial cells have a common origin. Because of the contractile nature of the myoepithelial cell, some workers have postulated a smooth muscle origin for these cells however most evidence suggests that both myoepithelial cells and epithelial cells arise from a common precursor cell, the 'clear' cell, basal B-cell or 'chief' cell (Vorherr, 1974) (Fig. 2.1).

The question of the cell of origin of breast epithelium is one of many that are potentially answerable using tissue culture methods. However, the breast has proved to be a difficult tissue to culture for many reasons. Firstly, many of its proliferative stages are under hormonal control, the components of which are still incompletely understood (Topper & Freeman, 1980). Secondly, the other nutritional requirements of human epithelial cells for in vitro growth are still being determined and mention will be made later of the role of growth factors in the in vitro growth of these cells. Thirdly, breast tissue has proved very difficult to disaggregate, because of the intermingling of epithelial and fibrous elements. Many methods have been developed to overcome this problem but none are completely satisfactory.

Culture methods

The culture of malignant and non-malignant (normal and hyperplastic) breast tissue will be considered separately but firstly some of the most commonly used methods will be considered.

Organ culture
Organ culture techniques rely on the ability of nutrients to perfuse into small pieces of tissue which retain their structural integrity. The method is limited as it is difficult to judge the success of a culture without using histological techniques. However, it has the advantage that the inter-relationship that exists

between epithelium and stroma is maintained. Although there are relatively few studies of normal mammary tissue in organ culture (Barker et al, 1964; Wellings & Jentoft, 1972), a recent study (Strum & Hillman, 1981) has demonstrated how this technique can be used to study the hormonal responses of normal mammary tissue.

An adaptation of the organ culture technique has been to grow small pieces of breast tissue or partially digested ductal elements in a three dimensional matrix (normally rat tail collagen). This technique has been applied with some success to studies on the morphogenesis of mammary glands [Emerman & Pitelka, 1977; Foster et al, 1983]).

Tissue culture

The term tissue culture is used to describe any method of growing individual cells without the constraints of the organisation of the tissue. Thus most tissue culture studies involve the growth of cells in two dimensions as a monolayer on a specially prepared surface. The initial problems faced when using this method are the disaggregation of the tissue and especially, the vexing problem of separating the epithelial cells from the stromal cells. Many attempts have been made to overcome these problems and procedures for the isolation of single cells have included both mechanical disruption techniques such as the 'spillage' technique of Lasfargues and Ozzello (1958) and complex enzyme digestion techniques. The most useful enzymes for disrupting mammary tissue while still maintaining the viability of the epithelial cells have been found to be collagenase and hyaluronidase. Digestion of normal breast tissue with these enzymes leads to the release of multicellular fragments of ducts and alveoli. These epithelial structures are stripped of stromal cells and basement membranes but because they retain their normal topology they are commonly referred to as organoids (Stampfer et al, 1980; Easty et al, 1981). In general digestion for periods of 18–24 hours at 37°C is necessary for good disaggregation (Easty et al, 1981; Biran et al, 1983).

Some workers have utilised an alternate approach to obtain mammary epithelial cells by making use of the fact that both ductal and lobular cells are shed into milk, especially in the post-weaning period (Buehring, 1972; Furmanski et al, 1974).

A further alternative to disaggregation is to use an explant culture technique. In this method, the tissue is dissected free of fat and obvious stroma and then cut into 1 mm cubes with a sharp scalpel. These small pieces are then placed in a minimal volume of medium. This is important as, if the medium volume is too great, the explants tend to float and the attachment which is necessary for outgrowth does not occur. The major problem with explant culture techniques (and with most other breast culture methods) is the overgrowth of the epithelial cells by fibroblastic cells arising from the stroma. It has been reported recently that removal of the explant tissue at days 10–14 eliminates the problem of fibroblast contamination (Whitehead & Brown, 1984).

The choice of culture medium for the growth of breast epithelial cells is still a matter of personal preference. Most systems use to date have comprised one of the commercially available tissue culture media (M199, Dulbecco's modification of Eagles Medium, RPMI 1640, Ham's F10, Leibowitz L15) plus foetal calf serum. As well as acting as a protein source, foetal calf serum also contains hormones such as oestrogen and progesterone (although these levels can vary widely from batch to batch) and other less well-defined growth and attachment factors. The use of other additives has varied but most workers are agreed that insulin is an essential growth factor for mammary tissue (Cailleau, 1973).

The need for other factors such as epidermal growth factor and cholera toxin is still uncertain although some workers support their use. The medium which we have found most satisfactory for the growth of both normal and malignant breast tissue is RPMI 1640 supplemented with 10% foetal calf serum, 0.6 μg/ml insulin, 1 μg/ml hydrocortisone, 10^{-5}M α-thioglycerol, 50 μg/ml penicillin and 50 units/ml streptomycin (Rowbottom et al, 1981; Whitehead et al, 1983). This medium has supported the growth of all human breast carcinoma cell lines and is also satisfactory for the initiation of growth of normal mammary epithelial cells from explant cultures.

The use of a variable ingredient such as foetal calf serum has rendered the study of the growth requirements of mammary cells almost impossible. The undefined hormonal content of this serum also makes hormonal studies impossible without such manoeuvres as hormone stripping with activated charcoal. The problem with this is that many other factors are removed by this procedure. There is therefore a great need for defined culture systems in which the requirement for serum has been replaced by defined components. Although a completely defined medium is not yet available Hammond, Ham and Stampfer (1983) have recently described a medium comprising MCDB 170 supplemented with 25 ng/ml epidermal growth factor, 0.5 μg/ml hydrocortisone, 5 μg/ml insulin and 0.1 mM each of ethanolamine and phosphoethanolamine. This medium would support the clonal growth of mammary cells if 7 μg/ml of a whole bovine pituitary extract was added. Although this factor is undefined it can be readily seen that this medium is a great advance over previous media.

Tissue culture studies

Normal mammary tissue

It is difficult to obtain normal mammary tissue from young healthy women, the best source being reduction mammoplasty material or the cells isolated from breast milk.

All studies of normal mammary tissue agree that two morphological types of epithelial cells can be cultured from normal mammary tissue. These cells have been designated E and E' cells and are illustrated in Figure 2.2. E cells are elongated flat cells growing in patches with distinct margination. E' cells are small cuboidal cells often with small vacuoles in the cytoplasm. Since the original description of milk as a source of epithelial cells (Buehring, 1972), a number of workers have used this system to study the growth of normal mammary cells in vitro. Hallowes et al (1977) cultured 65 lacteal secretions

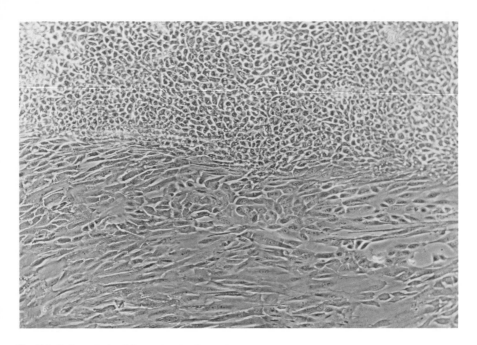

Fig. 2.2 Culture derived from a benign breast lesion. Both E'-type (top and E-type (bottom) cells are present in this culture (×90).

obtained either late in pregnancy or early in lactation and obtained growth of epithelial cells from 52 samples in dishes coated with rat-tail collagen. All of the cells cultured in this study were E-type cells. In contrast, Kirkland et al (1979) cultured cells from post-weaning milk and obtained cultures of both types of cell, often from the same donor. Recently Stoker, Perryman and Eeles (1982) have attempted to determine the inter-relationship of these cell types using a clonal assay system.

Studies using breast tissue from biopsy specimens have yielded similar cell types. Flaxman (1974) dissected out large ducts and digested small pieces with a trypsin-ethylene diamine tetracetic acid solution. All of the cultures were short term, but he described ultrastructural evidence for possible involvement of both epithelial and myoepithelial cells in his cultures.

Fibroblast contamination is always a problem with this type of system and the stimulation of fibroblast growth has been attributed to the presence of fetal calf serum in the medium. As mentioned previously a defined medium has recently been developed (Hammond et al, 1983). An alternate approach has been to replace the serum with high density lipoprotein and to use culture vessels coated with an extra-cellular matrix to aid cell adhesion (Biran et al, 1983). These culture conditions are reported to yield reliable epithelial growth from all biopsies cultures (Biran et al, 1983). If this can be repeated in other laboratories this will be a significant advance over all other culture methods previously described.

Collagen gels have also been used successfully for the culture of normal mammary epithelial tissue. This system has been used to study the proliferative potential of resting breast tissue (Foster et al, 1983). Using ^{3}H-thymidine pulse techniques these workers were able to demonstrate that approximately 10% of cells in the cultured organoids were proliferating 5 days after the initiation of culture. In addition, ultrastructural studies showed that the proliferating cells expressed neither epithelial nor myoepithelial features suggesting again that both epithelial and myoepithelial cells have a common precursor cell.

Benign breast disease tissue

One of the problems confronting workers attempting to culture tissue from benign lesions of the breast is the wide diversity of diseases encompassed by this classification (Azzopardi, 1979). The culture of cells from these lesions offers the potential for determining the cell of origin of these lesions.

A study of the growth of 21 fibroadenoma and nine benign mammary dysplasia lesions yielded growth of E-type cells in 95% of cases with E'-type cells being present in only one fibroadenoma culture (Hallowes et al, 1977). A similar study (Stoker, Pigott and Taylor-Papadimitriou, 1976) obtained short term growth of E-type cells with a doubling time of 2 days. However islands of cells ceased growing after reaching a maximum size of about 10^5 cells. This study demonstrated some growth enhancement of these cells by epidermal growth factor but failed to show any stimulation by oestradiol. The increases in growth shown were small compared to those induced by serum. A recent study of 86 benign biopsies showed that using a simple explant culture technique 76 (88%) yielded epithelial growth for at least 4 weeks and of these 59 were pure epithelial cultures free of fibroblasts. A further study in which the type of benign lesion was compared with the morphological cell type cultured showed that, as found previously, E-type cells predominated in cultures from fibroadenomas. In contrast biopsies of benign mammary dysplasia yielded mixed cultures of E'-type and E-type cells (Whitehead and Brown, 1984).

The availability of a technique which reliably yields sufficient cells which can be passaged has allowed us to study the nature of the E-type and E'-type cells in more detail. Using electron microscopy to investigate the ultrastructure of the cells and antibodies specific for the intracellular fibres, keratin, vimentin and myosin it has been shown that E-type cells have many of the characteristics (Table 2.1) of myoepithelial cells (Fig. 2.3) whereas E'-type cells resemble ductal epithelial cells (Whitehead et al, 1985) This finding suggests that E-type cells might either by myoepithelial in origin or arise from the common precursor cell with subsequent differentiation along the myoepithelial pathway. Studies such as these are important in increasing our understanding of the basic biology

Table 2.1 Markers distinguishing epithelial cells from myoepithelial.

Cell Type	Keratin	Vimentin	Myosin	MFGP*
Small, cuboidal epithelium (E')	+	+	−	+
Flatter, elongated cell (E)	+	+	+	+
Fibroblasts	−	+	+	−

* milk fat globule protein

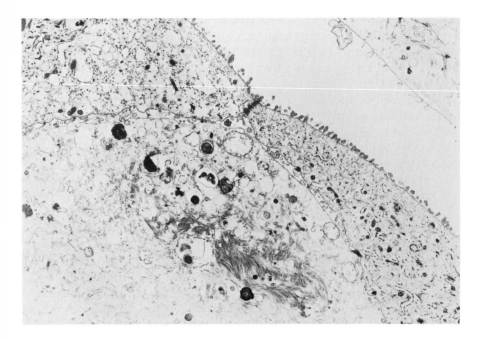

Fig. 2.3 Electron micrograph of cultured cells derived from a benign breast lesion. Epithelial cells with multiple microvilli and typical epithelial junctional complexes overlying a cell with multiple fibre bundles. This arrangement is typical of the arrangement seen in the breast. [Photograph supplied by Dr. P. Monaghan, Ludwig Institute for Cancer Research, London. Used by permission.] (×4550)

of benign breast lesions and are one way in which tissue culture techniques can contribute to our knowledge of breast pathology.

Breast carcinoma cultures

The culture of breast carcinoma cells has proved to be one of the most frustrating undertakings in tissue culture. In a pioneering work Cameron and Chambers (1937) described the outgrowth of epithelial cells from explants with subsequent overgrowth of fibroblasts. This has remained the central problem facing those who attempt to culture primary tumours and many methods have been described that attempt to overcome the problem of fibroblast contamination. Cameron and Chambers (1937) observed that the epithelial cells in their cultures did not adhere as tightly to the culture surface. This was substantiated by Cowman (1942, 1944) who described cultures with loose aggregates of cells with diminished cohesiveness.

Attempts at disaggregating breast tumours using conventional techniques such as mincing, yielded cell suspensions with a higher percentage of fibroblasts than epithelial cells (Whitescarver et al, 1968). From experiences such as this, Lasfargues and Ozzello (1958) developed a culture technique utilising only those cells which spilled freely from sliced tumour tissue and were successful in obtaining the first human breast carcinoma cell line, BT20. Originally this cell line required a very rich medium with many supplements for growth but with continual passage the growth requirements became less stringent until the cells would grow on conventional tissue culture media. It should be noted however that even using this technique these workers and many others since have failed to obtain further breast carcinoma cell lines from primary tumours. This suggests that the success of these workers (and others since) has depended on obtaining the right specimen rather than using the right technique. The problem with the spillage technique as with all others has been the contamination of cultures with fibroblasts and there is as yet no successful method of removing these contaminating cells from a culture.

Because of the problem of fibroblast contamination many workers have turned to metastatic disease sites and particularly to malignant effusions as a source of tumour cells for culture studies (Cailleau et al, 1974). Although fibroblasts are usually absent from this material the reactive mesothelial cell can cause problems (Whitehead & Hughes, 1975). In spite of this more breast carcinoma cell lines have been derived from this type of material than any other (MCF7, Soule et al, 1973; ZR-75-1, ZR-75-27, ZR-75-31, Engel et al, 1978; T47D, Keydar et al, 1979; PMC42, Whitehead et al, 1983a).

The availability of cell lines of malignant breast tumour cells has opened many avenues of study that were previously limited by a lack of sufficient tissue. It had long been recognised clinically that many breast tumours were hormonally dependent and although this had been exploited clinically the mechanism remained poorly understood. The finding therefore that one of the early breast carcinoma cell lines, MCF7, was responsive to oestrogen and contained oestrogen receptors (Brooks et al, 1973) gave rise to a large number of studies on the mechanisms of hormone action (Osborn & Lippman, 1978; Lippman, 1981) and in more recent times to studies on the mechanism of action of the anti-oestrogens such as tamoxiphen (Sutherland and Taylor, 1981).

Although it has been relatively easy to demonstrate the presence of hormone receptors on some of these cell lines it has proved much more difficult to identify biologically significant responses in these cell lines to the addition of the hormone. Because of difficulties in demonstrating proliferative responses of the breast tumour cell lines to oestrogen many of the studies have described the effects of hormones on the oestrogen and progesterone receptor machinery. It is only recently that ZR-75-1 cells have been reported to proliferate in a reproducible manner following the addition of oestrogen (Darbre, 1983).

The only breast carcinoma cell line that has receptors for both oestrogen and progesterone is PMC42 (Whitehead et al, 1983). This cell line will not proliferate in serum-free medium but will proliferate in response to the addition of oestrogen or progesterone to this medium. The response to the addition of both hormones is more than additive suggesting an enhancement of receptor numbers under these conditions (Whitehead et al, 1984). This cell line is also of interest because it appears to have retained the ability to differentiate under hormonal stimulus in vitro. Morphologically the cells are very heterogenous (Fig. 2.4) and 8 morphological cell types have been described and a differentiation pathway proposed (Whitehead et al, 1983a). In

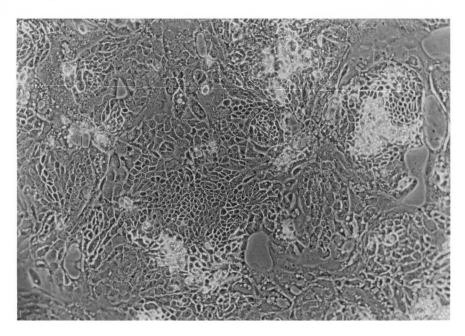

Fig. 2.4 Culture of PMC42 breast carcinoma cells showing the heterogeneity in the morphology of these cells (×90).

addition to growing as a monolayer the cells also grow as floating organoids with many of the cells resembling ductal cells morphologically and ultrastructurally. As mentioned above, the cells are responsive to hormones and in addition to the proliferative responses referred to, the cells synthesise and store lipid in response to the addition of prolactin at physiological levels (Whitehead et al, 1983b). The cells also respond to the addition of epidermal growth factor in a number of ways: the morphology of the cultured cells changes and many large cells appear in the culture; the growth rate of the cells and the cloning efficiency of the cells in semi-solid agar increases; the cells synthesise lipid and glycogen and deposit basement membrane proteins in the intracellular spaces. These findings involve both proliferation and differentiation and this is the only breast cancer cell line which responds to either prolactin or epidermal growth factor. As this cell line mimics the known hormonal responses of breast tissue (Topper & Freeman, 1970) in a way not found in any other cell line it has potential in many areas of breast physiology. In addition, the morphological heterogeneity and the apparent progression of one cell type to another suggest that the changes occurring in this cell line may represent the differentiation changes in normal breast as the putative stem cell differentiates into epithelial and myoepithelial cells. Although no overt myoepithelial cells have been identified in cultures of PMC42 it is of interest that two monoclonal antibodies raised against PMC42 cells stain only myoepithelial cells in normal breast tissue (Dempsey et al, to be published).

Neither this cell line nor any other breast cancer cell line described to the present has been shown to be capable of synthesising milk proteins such as casein or α-lactalbumin. Thus it would appear that the changes involved in the malignant process block the subsequent full differentiation of these cells. Therefore, although cell lines derived from breast carcinomas may be useful in many studies of the malignant process and even of the physiology of the breast there is still the need for the development of long term cultures of normal breast tissue which will be even more suitable for these studies. This remains a goal for future tissue culture studies.

In conclusion although it is only possible at present to culture normal and benign disease breast tissue for short periods this is sufficient for many studies. The culture of primary breast carcinomas is hindered by the proliferation of fibroblasts in most cultures. This type of culture is important however if we are to study the initial lesions in malignancy and the role of carcinogens and oncogenes in the malignant process. However, until better culture methods are developed, cell lines derived from metastatic deposits and especially malignant effusions will remain the mainstay of laboratory studies of breast cancer. It is hoped that the development of cell lines which retain more of the features of breast tissue than the anaplastic cell lines do, will enable us to advance our knowledge of the physiology of the breast and of the possible interactions of hormones and cytotoxic agents in breast cancer therapy. It is in systems such as this that tissue culture is a powerful tool and there will be increasing exploitation of the potential of this system in the years ahead.

Alternate techniques

Because of the difficulty of growing normal mammary epithelium there have been attempts to obtain permanent cell lines by transforming primary cells with known oncogenic viruses (Chang et al, 1982). These workers found that although it was easy to transform breast epithelial cells with SV40 virus, most of the transformed cells eventually died out. However they did obtain one continuous line of transformed cells which retained breast markers on the cell membrane.

At alternate approach to the proliferation of breast carcinoma tissue has been to implant the tissue either into nude, congenitally athymic mice (Rae-Venter and Reid, 1980) or into thymectomised, whole body irradiated, bone marrow reconstituted mice (Bailey et al, 1981). It is interesting to note that even in these animal systems some breast carcinomas require hormone supplements for growth (Leung & Shiv, 1981).

REFERENCES

Azzopardi J G 1979 Problems in breast pathology. W B Saunders and Co, London
Bailey M J, Ormerod M G, Imrie S F, Humphreys J, Roberts J D B, Gazet J-C, Neville A M 1981 Comparative functional histopathology of human breast carcinoma xenografts. British Journal of Cancer 43: 125–134
Barker B E, Fanger H, Farnes P 1964 Human mammary slices in organ culture. I Method of culture and preliminary observations on the effect of insulin. Experimental Cell Research 35: 437–448

Biran S, Horowitz A T, Fuks Z, Vlodavsky I 1983 High density lipoprotein and extracellular matrix promotes growth and plating efficiency of normal human mammary epithelial cells in serum-free medium. International Journal of Cancer 31: 557–566

Brooks S C, Locke E R, Soule H D 1973 Estrogen receptor in a human cell line (MCF7) from breast carcinoma. Journal of Biological Chemistry 248: 6251–6253

Buehring G C 1972 Culture of human mammary epithelial cells: Keeping abreast with a new method. Journal of the National Cancer Institute 49: 1433–1434

Cailleau R 1973 Old and new problems in human tumor cell cultivation. In: Fogh J (ed) Human tumor cells in vitro. Plenum Press, New York. p 79–114

Cailleau R, Mackay B, Young R K, Reeves W J 1974 Tissue culture studies on pleural effusions from breast carcinoma patients. Cancer Research 34: 801–809

Cameron G, Chambers R 1937 Neoplasm studies. iii Organization of cells of human tumors in tissue culture. American Journal of Cancer 30: 115–129

Chang S E, Keen J, Lane E B, Taylor-Papadimitriou J 1982 Establishment and characterization of SV40-transformed human breast epithelial cell lines. Cancer Research 42: 2040–2053

Cowman D R 1942 Human neoplasms in tissue culture. Cancer Research 2: 618–625

Cowman D R 1944 Decreased mutual adhesiveness, a property of cells from squamous cell carcinomas. Cancer Research 4: 625–629

Darbre P, Yates J, Curtis S, King R J B 1983 Effect of estradiol on human breast cancer cells in culture. Cancer Research 43: 349–354

Easty G C, Easty D M, Monaghan P, Ormerod M G, Neville A M 1981 Preparation and identification of human breast epithelial cells in culture. International Journal of Cancer 26: 577–584

Emerman J T, Pitelka D R 1977 Maintenance and induction of morphological differentiation of dissociated mammary epithelium on floating collagen membranes. In Vitro 13: 316–328

Engel L W, Young N A, Tralka T S, Lippman M E, O'Brein S J, Joyce M 1978 Establishment and characterization of three new continuous cell lines derived from human breast carcinomas. Cancer Research 38: 3352–3364

Foster C S, Smith C A, Dinsdale E A, Monaghan P, Munro Neville A 1983 Human mammary gland morphogenesis in vitro: The growth and differentiation of normal breast epithelium in collagen gel cultures defined by electron microscopy, monoclonal antibodies, and autoradiography. Developmental Biology 96: 197–216

Flaxman B A 1974 In vitro studies of the normal human mammary gland. Journal of Investigative Dermatology 63: 48–57

Furmanski P, Longley C, Fouchey D, Rich R, Rich M A 1974 Normal human mammary cells in culture: Evidence for onconavirus-like particles. Journal of the National Cancer Institute 52: 975–977

Hallowes R C, Millis R, Pigott D, Shearer M, Stoker M G P, Taylor-Papadimitriou J 1977 Results on a pilot study of cultures of human lacteal secretions and benign and malignant breast tumours. Clinical Oncology 3: 81–90

Hammond S L, Ham R G, Stampfer M R 1983 Rapid clonal growth and serial passage of normal human mammary epithelial cells in a defined medium. Proceedings of the International Association for Breast Cancer Research p 59

Keydar I, Chen L, Karby S, Weiss F R, Delarea J, Radu M, Chaitcik S, Brenner W J 1979 Establishment and characterization of a cell line of human breast carcinoma origin. European Journal of Cancer 15: 659–670

Kirkland W L, Yang N-S, Jorgensen T, Longley C, Furmanski P 1979 Growth of normal and malignant human mammary epithelial cells in culture. Journal of the National Cancer Institute 63: 29–41

Lasfargues E Y, Ozzello L 1958 Cultivation of human breast carcinomas. Journal of the National Cancer Institute 21: 1131–1147

Leung C K H, Shiv P C 1981 Required presence of both estrogen and pituitary factors for the growth of human breast cancer cells in athymic nude mice. Cancer Research 41: 546–551

Lippman M 1981 Hormonal regulation in human breast cancer cells in vitro. Banbury Reports 8: 171–181

Osborn C K, Lippman M E 1978 Human breast cancer in tissue culture: the effects of hormones. In: McGuire W L (ed) Breast Cancer: Advances in Research and Treatment Volume 2. Plenum Press, New York p 103–154

Rae-Venter B, Reid L M 1980 Growth of human breast carcinomas in nude mice and subsequent establishment in tissue culture. Cancer Research 40: 95–100

Rowbottom L A, Whitehead R H, Roberts G P, Hughes L E 1981 A study of the growth requirements of human tumour cells in tissue culture. Australian Journal of Experimental Biology and Medical Science 59: 91–100

Soule H D, Vazquez J, Long A, Albert S, Brennan M 1973 A human cell line from a pleural effusion derived from a breast carcinoma. Journal of the National Cancer Institute 51: 1409–1416

Stampfer M R, Hallowes R C, Hackett A J 1980 Growth of normal mammary cells in culture. In Vitro 26: 415–425

Stoker M, Perryman M, Eeles R 1982 Clonal analysis of morphological phenotype in cultured mammary epithelial cells from human milk. Proceedings of the Royal Society, London B215: 231–240

Stoker M G P, Pigott D, Taylor-Papamitriou J 1976 Response to epidermal growth factors of cultured human mammary epithelial cells from benign tumours. Nature 264: 764–767

Strum J M, Hillman E A 1981 Human breast epithelium in organ culture: Effect of hormones on growth and morphology. In Vitro 17: 33–43

Sutherland R L, Taylor D W 1981 Effect of tamoxifen on the cell cycle kinetics of cultured human mammary carcinoma cells. Reviews on Endocrine-Related Cancer, Supplement 8: 17–25

Topper Y J, Freeman C S 1980 Multiple hormone interactions in the developmental biology of the mammary gland. Physiological Reviews 60: 1049–1106

Vorherr H 1974 The Breast. Morphology, Physiology and Lactation. Academic Press, New York

Wellings S R, Jentoft V L 1972 Organ culture of normal, dysplastic, hyperplastic and neoplastic human mammary tissues. Journal of the National Cancer Institute 49: 329–338

Whitehead R H, Bertoncello I, Webber L M, Pedersen J S 1983a A new human breast carcinoma cell line (PMC42) with stem cell characteristics. I. Morphological characterization. Journal of the National Cancer Institute 70: 649–661

Whitehead R H, Brown R W 1984 The culture of epithelial cells from benign breast lesions. International Journal of Breast and Mammary Pathology 2: 167–171

Whitehead R H, Hughes L E 1975 Tissue culture studies of malignant effusions. British Journal of Cancer 32: 512–518

Whitehead R H, Monaghan P, Webber L M, Bertoncello I, Vitali A A 1983b A new human breast carcinoma cell line (PMC42). II. Characterization of cells growing as organoids. Journal of the National Cancer Institute 71: 1193–1203

Whitehead R H, Quirk S J, Vitali A A, Funder J W, Sutherland R L, Murphy L C 1984 A new human breast carcinoma cell line (PMC 42) with stem cell characteristics. III. Hormonal receptor status and responsiveness. Journal of the National Cancer Institute 73: 643–648.

Whitehead R H, Pedersen J S, Monaghan P, Brown R W 1985 Detection of cells with epithelial and myoepithelial properties in cultures derived from benign breast disease. International Journal of Breast and Mammary Pathology (in press)

Whitescarver J, Recher L, Sykes J A, Briggs L 1968 Problems involved in culturing breast tissues. Texas Reports on Biology and Medicine 26: 613–628

3 The endocrine control of breast cancer

C. FRED LEMAISTRE and WILLIAM L. MCGUIRE

Introduction

The significance of the breast cancer problem is obvious, with over one million cases of breast cancer in women reported worldwide each year. The incidence of breast cancer continues to increase globally, especially in Western countries and in developing countries (Cutler et al, 1976). We may therefore expect the magnitude of the problem of breast cancer to grow.

It has long been recognized that the female reproductive organs have a role in the genesis of breast cancer. Bernardo Ramazzini (1713) commented on the 'mysterious sympathy' that exists between the female genital organs and the breast over two centuries ago. A century later, Rigoni Stern noted that the Catholic Sisters of Verona, Italy had an increased risk of breast cancer compared with non-monastic women (Clemmensen, 1951).

Recent epidemiologic studies have focused on the potential effect of endogenous and exogenous hormonal factors on the risk of developing breast cancer. Several hormonal factors have been identified that appear to alter a woman's risk of developing breast cancer (Table 3.1). Breast cancer has been found to be more common in single than in married women, to occur more frequently in nonparous than parous women and to be correlated with age of first pregnancy (Lilienfield, 1956; Logan, 1953; MacMahon et al, 1970; MacMahon et al, 1973). Analysis of the series of MacMahon demonstrated the single most important factor relating pregnancy to breast cancer is the age of the mother at first birth. This effect appears to induce irreversible changes

Table 3.1 Hormonally related factors that predispose to breast cancer

Prolonged menstrual activity—early menarche, late menopause
  Nulliparous or > 35 at 1st childbirth
  Progesterone deficit
  Postmenopausal weight

Hormonally related facts that protect against breast cancer
  First childbirth at < 20 years
  High parity
  Ovariectomy

such that the decreased risk is still found among women in their eighth and ninth decades. Pregnancy is characterized by a vast change in a variety of hormones. The protective effect of early pregnancy may be related to changes induced in the breast by these hormones rendering breast tissue less susceptible to carcinogenesis.

Prolonged exposure to endogenous estrogens may increase the risk of breast cancer. Woman with early menarche and with late age of menopause appear to be at increased risk for developing breast cancer (Zumoff et al, 1975; Kelsey, 1979). On the other hand, those women with early menopause appear to be afforded relative protection (Trichopoulos et al, 1972; Lilienfield, 1956; Feinleib, 1968). It has been suggested that estrogens may be particularly effective in increasing risk when unopposed by progesterone as in the follicular phase of the menstrual cycle or in cycles with a difficient luteal phase (Sherman & Korenman, 1974; Sherman et al, 1982). Korenman (1980) has further suggested that the predominant action of the unopposed estrogen would occur in the postmenarcheal years and in the pre and perimenopausal period when luteal deficient cycles are most frequent. This hypothesis would account for early menarche and late menopause as risk factors in breast cancer. A recent study in young women could not confirm this hypothesis as the duration of anovular cycles is the same for women with late or early menarche. There is also no evidence that the frequency of anovular cycles is higher in young women in areas where breast cancer risk is high (MacMohan et al, 1982).

There appears to be a firm relationship between obesity and risk for breast cancer (Hankin et al, 1978; de Waard et al, 1977). In postmenopausal women, the major source of estrogens is from the extraglandular conversion of androstendione to estrone. A principal site for this conversion is fat cells. Thus heavy women would be expected to have elevated estrogen levels.

If estrogens act as tumor promoters by increasing the growth of mammary ductal epitheal cells that are targets for whatever else causes breast cancer, then the role of exogenous steroid hormones in altering breast cancer risk assumes obvious importance. The evidence for the association of estrogens and oral contraceptives in the development of breast cancer has been extensively detailed (Drill, 1981; Thomas, 1982). A number of studies have been unable to demonstrate an increased risk for women taking oral contraceptives (Vessey et al, 1976; Vessey et al, 1972; Paffenbarger et al, 1977; Kelsey, 1979). Review of studies examining the risk of breast cancer in relation to replacement estrogens has generated some disagreement (Drill, 1981; Kelsey, 1979; Thomas, 1982). Moderate use of estrogens for menopausal symptoms probably has little effect on risk, but long term users and women who take high strength preparations may increase their risk. Moreover, exogenous estrogens may reduce the protective effect of premenopausal oophorectomy and may preferentially enhance the risk of breast cancer in women with some types of benign breast disease (Thomas, 1982). Published studies are only suggestive of increased risk in these subgroups and the interaction of estrogens with known risk factors, the importance of dose and duration of therapy deserve further study.

As breast cancer rarely occurs in the undeveloped breast, it is at least clear that these hormones are necessary for mammary gland growth. The presence of estrogens and progesterone serve to prepare the background for the action of genetic factors, viral and environmental factors in the initiation of malignancy. Once initiated, many breast tumors remain under hormonal control. The remainder of this chapter will review the role of steroid hormones in the biology and treatment of breast cancer.

Mechanism of action

Normal mammary tissue as well as its neoplastia possess receptors for a variety of steroid and peptide hormones. Because of their clinical utility in the management of breast cancer, the receptors for estrogen and progesterone have attracted the most interested.

In order to define the mechanism of action of steroid hormones, a number of investigators have established in vitro systems utilizing cell lines derived from human breast cancers. The MCF-7 cell line is probably among the best characterized of these cell lines and meets the criteria of karyology, protein phenotyping and differentiated function necessary to confirm its mammary origin (Soule et al, 1973; Russo et al, 1976, Knazek et al, 1977). Further, it contains receptors for a number of steroid hormones (Horwitz et al, 1975). While the direct application of in vitro hormonal effects to the clinical arena is fraught with hazzard (Lippman, 1981), we have gained new insights into hormone dependency.

The precise mechanism by which any steroid hormones induce gene activity and increases in metabolism in not known. Steroids freely cross the cell membrane and enter the target cell cytoplasm. In the case of estradiol, it is then bound by a cytoplasmic estrogen receptor (ER). The ER bind 17β estradiol with high affinity, but is also capable of binding other steroid hormones with lower affinity such as 17α estradiol, androgens, and anti-estrogens (Edwards & McGuire, 1980; Zava & McGuire, 1978; Horwitz and McGuire, 1980). Once bound, the ER undergoes important changes that enhance its ability to translocate to the nucleus (ERN) and to induce DNA transcription. These changes, characterized as 'nucleotropy' and 'activation', are thought to be independent (Jungblut et al, 1979). Neither the mechanism by which these changes are induced nor the resulting interaction are well understood. Some observers have suggested that the interaction between ligand and receptor produces a specific allosteric change (Bullock et al, 1978) and that differences in response to different steroids may be a result of such stereospecificity (Rochefort & Borgna, 1981).

In MCF-7 cells the estrogen-ER complex is translocated to the nucleus within minutes. The translocated nuclear receptor then undergoes rapid processing such that by 3–5 hours after binding, 70% or more of the ERN are lost from the cells without reappearance of unfilled sites (Horwitz & McGuire, 1980). The way in which ERN interacts with the DNA-histone complex has not been properly elucidated. Much later, the results of this interaction yield altered DNA function, the production of a multitude of proteins and effects on growth.

Estrogen administration increases net DNA synthesis in vitro in a time dependent fashion, a process modulated by the availability of thymidine. E_2 stimulated cells incorporate exogenous thymidine into their nuclei in preference to thymidine generated from intracellular salvage pathways, thus increasing intracellular thymidine pools (Lippman & Aitken, 1980). Estrogen stimulation also induces enzymes implicated in cell proliferation such as DNA polymerase α and enzymes involved in nucleotide salvage (Edwards & McGuire, 1980; Edwards et al, 1980; Bronzert et al, 1981). A host of other proteins modulated by estrogen have been detailed in a recent review (Adams et al, 1983) and are listed in Table 3.2.

Table 3.2 Estrogen regulation of specific proteins

Progesterone receptor
Lactate dehydrogenase
DNA polymerase alpha
Thymidine kinase
Endogenous peroxidase
Lactalbumin
Thiol protease
Plasminogen activator
46K ⎫
24K ⎬ Estrogen regulated proteins of unknown function (see Adams et al, 1983)
54K ⎭

Of all the protein products of estrogen regulated DNA transcription, the progesterone receptor has generated the most interest. It is now clear that the chances of successful endocrine therapy are greatly improved when estrogen receptor is present in a breast cancer. However, 30–40% of estrogen positive tumours will not respond leading to the concept that ER is a necessary, but not sufficient marker of endocrine responsiveness (Horwitz et al, 1975). Horwitz & McGuire (1978) have clearly demonstrated the induction of PgR in human breast cancer in vitro. Since estrogen receptor is only the initial step in a complex biochemical pathway, it is possible that in endocrine resistant, ER positive tumors lesions might exist in later steps concerned with hormone action. Therefore a product of hormone action such as PgR would be a better marker of hormone responsiveness. This observation appears to be clinically valid. Fisher et al (1983) examined the quantitative concordance of ER and PgR in 1887 patients with breast cancer. In this study only 13% of patients displayed PgR with an ER in the negative range. The fact that PgR is present in ER negative tumors has been a consistent finding, though usually accounting for 3–5% of tumors (Bloom et al, 1980; Young et al, 1980; McGuire & Horwitz, 1978). This discordance has evoked a number of technical and methodologic explanations (Edwards et al, 1979; Panko & McLeod, 1978; Zava et al, 1977). As will be discussed later, however, the presence of PgR also carries within it an improved prognosis and improved endocrine responsiveness.

Steroid receptors and prognosis

Measurement of steroid receptors

Of all the measurable steroid hormone receptors present in human breast neoplasia, interest has focused on the estrogen and progesterone receptors because of their clinical utility. The methodology for assaying these receptors has been extensively reviewed (Chamness & McGuire, 1979), therefore only a few general comments will be made.

Both estrogen and progesterone receptor are very unstable at room temperature making proper tissue handling critical to the reliability of the assay results. The biopsy sample should immediately be cooled on ice and sent to the pathologist. If the specimen is obtained during mastectomy, the tumor tissue should not remain in the mastectomy specimen until the completion of the procedure. Rather, an excisional biopsy should be performed and sent to the pathologist on ice. A delay of only minutes in cooling the tissue may result in a false negative result. Upon receipt of the specimen, the pathologist must trim the specimen of fat, normal tissue, and obvious necrosis as these tissues do not contain receptor and may contribute to a falsely low value. After trimming, the tumor must be frozen at once in liquid nitrogen or by quick freezing in the cryostat. The frozen tissue should be kept in dry ice avoiding 'frost free' freezers or cryostats with cyclic temperature fluctuations.

A number of established methods have been reported for the assay of steroid receptors (Chamness & McGuire, 1979). Receptor assay methodology has improved considerably in recent years and the sucrose density gradient centrifugation or dextran-coated charcoal techniques are the methods in most widespread use. Both methods provide reproducible results in trained hands.

The tissue is homogenized and the soluble receptor fraction is obtained by ultracentrifugation. A wide range of concentrations of ^{125}I-estradiol for ER analysis and ^{3}H-R5020 for PgR analysis are added to the soluble cytosol fraction, which contains the receptors. The bound and free radioactive steroids are then separated and nonradioactive competitors are used to measure nonspecific binding. Scatchard analysis is used to analyze the data so that precise quantitative results can be obtained. These are reported as femtomoles of receptor per milligram of cytosol protein.

Although the biochemical assay of these receptors is reliable, they are characterized by a number of inherent disadvantages. They require time and expensive equipment and they do not reveal which or how many of the tumor cells actually contain receptor. A number of investigators have pursued various histochemical and immunohistochemical techniques to obviate these disadvantages. Theoretically, a valid histochemical technique would permit assessment of all morphological features and additionally would be rapid, inexpensive, and could be performed on minute tissue samples. Unfortunately, in spite of their great potential, none of these procedures has yet been fully validated as detecting receptors (Chamness et al, 1980; Chamness & McGuire, 1982).

Steroid receptors and cellular differentiation

Independent of receptor status, survival of patients with breast cancer appears to be related to the degree of differentiation of the malignancy. Tumors that morphologically and metabolically most closely resemble normal breast epithelium usually have a more indolent course and better prognosis; less differentiated tumors tend to be more aggressive and are associated with poor patient survival. Thus, tumors with an histologic appearance reminiscent of normal breast structures such as tubular (Taylor & Norris, 1970) or mucinous (Norris & Taylor, 1965) subtypes have a more favorable prognosis than infiltrating ductal carcinoma not otherwise specified. Furthermore, tumor with less morphologic atypia (low histologic grade; high nuclear grade) have a better prognosis than more anaplastic tumors (Fisher, 1977; Bloom, 1950; Champion et al 1972).

A number of studies correlating primary breast cancer histopathology with ER content have demonstrated that ER negative tumors tend to be less well differentiated than ER positive tumors. The presence of ER is consistently associated with high nuclear and low histologic grades, absence of tumor necrosis, and presence of marked tumor elastosis (Antoniades & Spector, 1979; Fisher et al, 1981; Fisher et al, 1980; Hartveit et al, 1981; McCarty et al, 1980; Martin et al, 1979; Maynard et al, 1978; Millis, 1980; Rolland et al, 1980; Silfversward et al, 1980).

PgR status has also been correlated with certain pathologic features. Millis (1980) reported that well differentiated tumors were more frequently PgR positive than poorly differentiated tumors. McCarty et al (1980) observed the same relationship and noted that the relationship between receptor content and histologic grade was enhanced by considering ER and PgR simultaneously. Delarue et al (1981) demonstrated that a higher portion of inflammatory tumors are PgR negative than operable tumors.

Kinetic studies of breast tumors using either the thymidine labeling index or flow cytometry to estimate the S phase fraction correlate with histologic observations. ER negative tumors are more aneuploid than ER positive tumors (Muss et al, 1980; Kute et al, 1981) and have a higher labeling index (Meyer et al, 1977; Cooke et al, 1980; Gioanni et al, 1979). ER negative premenopausal patients have the highest proliferative activity (Bertuzzi et al, 1981a).

These studies would suggest that ER and PgR are biochemical markers for tumor differentiation. At present, however, it is unclear whether histologic and kinetic parameters of differentiation and receptor status are independent variables with a high degree of association or if one is dependent on the other for its expression.

Steroid receptors and prognosis

Based on cell kinetic and morphologic studies, human breast cancer may be conceptually divided into well differentiated, less aggressive, receptor positive tumours or less differentiated, more aggressive, receptor negative tumors. Clinical studies correlating disease free survival support this concept.

Knight et al (1977) were the first to demonstrate a significant difference in disease free interval after mastectomy using the ER. Patients whose tumor contained ER recurred less frequently than those whose tumor did not have ER, a finding which was independent of the size of the primary tumor, the number of involved lymph nodes, menopausal status or duration of adjuvant therapy. A subgroup that appeared to be at high risk of recurrence were those patients with involved axillary nodes and absence of ER in their tumor. Approximately half of these patients recurred within 18 months of surgery. Subsequent studies have confirmed these observations (Allegra & Lippman, 1980; Bertuzzi et al 1981a; Hartveit et al, 1980; Leake et al, 1980; Rich et al, 1978; Furmanski et al, 1980). As one might expect, the differences observed in disease free interval based on ER also translates into differences in survival (Bishop et al 1979; Gapinski & Donegan, 1980; Hahnel et al, 1979; Kinne et al, 1981; Samaan et al, 1981; Stewart et al, 1981). Of interest, the length of survival from recurrence does not correlate with quantitative receptor content but rather is dependent on whether the tumor was positive or negative.

Although not all investigators agree, there appears to be a correlation between the ER status of the primary tumor and subsequent patterns of metastasis (Hahnel et al, 1979; Walt et al, 1976; Shinghakowinata et al, 1976; Stewart et al, 1981; Campbell et al, 1981). Current evidence suggests that ER negative tumors are more likely to recur as a metastasis in visceral organs such as brain or liver, thereby causing increased morbidity and mortality. On the other hand, ER positive tumors not only seem to metastasize less readily, but are more likely to spread to bone than viscera.

The presence of PgR also predicts for an improved disease free survival. As has been discussed, there is good rationale for this relationship because the synthesis of PgR is dependent on estrogen stimulation in normal reproductive tissues and human breast cancer cell lines in culture and because the presence of PgR correlates with histologically well differentiated tumors that have low thymidine labeling indices. Since the presence of ER predicts for improved survival one might expect that patients whose tumors possess PgR may constitute a prognostically superior group. In fact, this appears to be the case as several investigators have found the presence of PgR in a tumor to be of positive prognostic value. Saez et al (1981) examined the prognostic value of ER and PgR in patients with resectable breast cancer and found the recurrence rate for patients with both receptors was significantly less than for patients who lacked these receptors. Pinchon et al (1980) investigated the relationship between PgR and prognosis in a small group of patients with various stages of early breast cancer and concluded that those patients whose tumor contained PgR experienced a markedly lower rate of metastases. These findings are in accord with those of Bertuzzi, Vezzoni & Ronchi (1981b) who found PgR to be a better discriminating recurrence than ER for node negative patients.

Investigators at our institution have also recently examined the prognostic value of PgR in patients with primary breast cancer (Clark et al, 1983). 318 women with stage II breast cancer underwent radical or modified radical mastectomies and were randomly assigned to receive one of three adjuvant treatment modalities: chemotherapy alone or chemotherapy plus hormonal therapy with or without BCG. As expected, the number of positive axillary nodes was the most important predictor of disease free survival. The presence of PgR was the second most important predictor of disease free survival and actually surpassed ER in its capacity to predict time to recurrence. In other words, if the number of positive nodes, tumor size, and PgR content of the tumor are known, the ER levels did not enhance the prediction of recurrence.

Prognostic studies, such as those mentioned, have important therapeutic and experimental implications. It is of obvious important that clinical studies comparing treatment regimens should stratify patients by estrogen and progesterone receptor status, just as is currently done for nodal status and other prognostic factors. Moreover, knowledge of such prognostic factors should be used to guide the design of new treatment strategies. For example, patients whose tumors are receptor negative and involve axillary nodes may be the most important target for aggressive adjuvant therapy because of their poor prognosis. On the other hand, receptor positive node negative patients may well be spared the rigors of adjuvant therapy because of the favorable prognosis.

Steroid hormones and therapy of breast cancer

That tumor regression of breast cancer may be achieved with endocrine manipulation was first observed almost a century ago (Schinzinger, 1889; Beatson, 1896). Systematic exploitation of surgical ablative procedures was pursued in this century, but the disappointing results of prophylactic ablative measures lead to their application in advanced disease (Taylor, 1939; Huggins & Bergenstal, 1951; Huggins & Dao, 1954; Horsley & Horsley, 1962; Nissen Meyer, 1964; Kennedy et al, 1964). Surgical ablation of endocrine organs was found to produce clinical responses in less than a third of patients, more commonly in postmenopausal women and in women with a long disease free interval after primary surgery.

The clinical criteria used to select patients for hormonal therapy in these studies were (and still are) imprecise. The discovery of the ER provided an improved understanding of which tumors would respond to hormonal therapies (McGuire et al, 1975). These findings have been amplified in recent years and collectively emphasize the need for steroid receptor analysis in all cases of breast cancer.

The improved understanding of receptor physiology (reviewed earlier in this chapter) has enhanced the clinicians ability to identify potentially endocrine sensitive tumors. It is important to recognize, however, that the mechanism by which hormones affect the growth and behavior of breast neoplasia is not known. While the estrogen receptor pathway is clearly a marker of endocrine sensitivity, there is no evidence that the various endocrine therapeutic modalities act through this pathway. Further, it is not clear whether these modalities induce cellular differentiation and inhibition of cell division or whether they are directly cytotoxic.

When planning appropriate endocrine therapy of breast cancer certain observations are now accepted as basic. Less than 10% of women with ER negative tumors will respond to hormonal therapy. Conversely only 50–60% of patients with ER positive tumors will respond to endocrine manipulation. If one postulates that the presence of PgR is indicative of a complete receptor pathway, one might expect that it will be a more effective predictor of endocrine responsives. This appears to be the case as patients whose tumors possess both receptors respond more frequently than those containing only one or no receptor (Osborne et al, 1980; Degenshein et al, 1980; Clark & McGuire, 1983). Apparently a biologically intact receptor pathway is necessary for successful hormonal manipulation.

A bewildering array of modalities are available for hormonal manipulation of endocrine responsive tumors. For simplicity these may be divided into ablative and additive therapies (Table 3.3). The preferred utilization of these alternatives in advanced disease has recently been received by Osborne & McGuire (1983). Rather than reiterate these concepts we will focus on hormonal therapy as it pertains to early breast cancer.

Table 3.3 Ablative therapies

Surgical ablation
  Ovariectomy
  Adrenalectomy
  Hypophysectomy
Medical ablation
  Medical adrenalectomy (aminoglutethimide)
Additive therapies
  Estrogens
  Androgens
  Progestins
  Corticosteroids
  Antiestrogens (tamoxifen)

Adjuvant hormonal therapy in early breast cancer

There is little question that both cytoxic chemotherapy and endocrine therapy can cause dramatic regression of advanced breast cancer. Less dramatic is the impact of these modalities on overall survival, reinforcing the importance of the observed delay in relapse and prolonged survival seen in some patients following adjuvant chemotherapy for early breast cancer.

Since Schinzinger first suggested that oophorectomy was useful in the containment of breast cancer in 1889, nearly twenty trials have been published examining this therapy. Most of these studies have examined ovarian ablation either through surgical castration or ovarian irradiation. It is still not clear if adjuvant ovarian ablation is useful because of poor study design, small numbers of patients, and the absence of receptor data in these studies.

The first prospective trial of 'prophylactic' ovarian ablation using irradiation was undertaken in premenopausal patients in Manchester. Although the 5 and 7 year relapse rates were significantly different untreated versus untreated patients the delay in relapse occurred in the first year after mastectomy (Cole, 1970). A second such trial conducted in Norway led to the conclusion that in primarily castrated patients the disease free survival was increased in both pre and postmenopausal patients (Nissen Meyer, 1964). In this study there appeared to be no advantage to castration by surgery over castration by irradiation.

Nevinny et al (1969) reported the first controlled trial of adjuvant oophorectomy. The survival benefit at the time of report was marginal and the authors concluded there was no overall benefit. This was supported by the report of the National Surgical Adjuvant Breast Project, NSABP, (Ravdin et al 1970) although the numbers of patients in both trials was small.

A further trial was reported from Canada examining the effect of prophylatic radiation menopause with or without prednisolone on relapse and survival (Meakin et al, 1979). In premenopausal patients who received ovarian irradiation, the recurrence of breast cancer was delayed and survival prolonged, but not significantly so. A significantly delayed recurrence and survival advantage was seen in premenopausal women receiving ovariation irradiation plus prednisolone. Whether the prednisolone produced this effect by suppressing adrenal production of estrogen is not known. Ovarian irradiation with or without prednisolone was demonstrated to be of no value in postmenopausal patients.

Finally, there is one uncontrolled report in 17 postmenopausal patients with four or more positive axillary nodes suggesting a significant extension of survival (Dao et al, 1975). It is clinically difficult to propose a large scale trial to evaluate adjuvant adrenalectomy, although 'medical adrenalectomy' with aminoglutethimide provides a rational alternative to examine this question.

In the last decade, additive endocrine treatment with the antiestrogen tamoxifen has caused renewed interest in adjuvant hormonal therapy. This agent avoids the morbidity associated with ovarian ablation and lacks the undesirable side effects of androgens and estrogens. Several trials are underway at present examining the benefit of tamoxifen in the adjuvant setting. From the study of Brinkley & Haybittle (1975), it is clear that prolonged follow-up is critical to the interpretation of any study examining adjuvant therapy. Although many of the trials examining adjuvant tamoxifen are not yet 'mature', some interesting observations have been made.

The first study examining adjuvant tamoxifen compared the contribution of tamoxifen, with or without immunotherapy to adjuvant chemotherapy (Hubay et al 1981). Patients with stage II breast cancer were randomized to receive either a combination of cytoxan, methotrexate and 5-fluorouracil (CMF) or CMF plus tamoxifen for one year or CMF plus tamoxifen plus BCG vaccination. ER status was known and in ER negative patients, there was no significant differences in relapse rate. In patients with ER positive tumors, there was a lower relapse rate for CMF plus tamoxifen compared to CMF alone. The addition of BCG did not alter this finding. The early results of this study indicate that tamoxifen plus chemotherapy is more effective in delaying recurrence than chemotherapy alone in patients with ER positive stage II breast cancer.

In Manchester a large controlled trial has been undertaken examining tamoxifen as an adjuvant treatment of early breast cancer. After primary treatment, premenopausal patients were randomized to receive either irradiation menopause or tamoxifen for one year while postmenopausal patients received either tamoxifen or placebo (Riberio & Palmer, 1983). Although the trial is still early, there appears to be no difference between tamoxifen and irradiation menopause in premenopausal patients. In postmenopausal patients, overall survival was not significantly influenced by tamoxifen, with the exception of these patients with four or more involved axillary nodes. Unfortunately, receptor data was not included in the trial.

In Copenhagen, premenopausal patients were randomized after primary therapy to receive tamoxifen for 2 years or placebo, while postmenopausal patients were additionally randomized to DES (Palshoff, 1981). The recurrence rate in premenopausal patients was lower in patients receiving tamoxifen. Surprisingly, those premenopausal patients with ER negative tumors recurred less frequently than those whose tumors were ER positive. In postmenopausal patients, the recurrence rate was reduced in the groups receiving either DES or tamoxifen compared with placebo. This finding was correlated with the presence of ER. The findings from this preliminary report should be viewed cautiously as patients were treated by simple mastectomy and axillary nodes status, a critical prognostic factor, was not known. Further, there was a high incidence (58%) of ER negative tumors compared with other series and in premenopausal patients this was an unexpectedly and apparently favorable prognosis.

A number of other trials examining adjuvant tamoxifen are ongoing in the Eastern Cooperative oncology Group, Ludwig Breast Cancer Study Group, DBCCG and United Kingdom. All are at early stages and the studies must mature for meaningful interpretation.

Finally, the NSABP has reported the initial findings from their study randomizing women with stage II breast cancer to either melphalan and 5 fluorouracil (PF) with or without tamoxifen (PFT) (Fisher et al 1983a). The overall results at 3 years show that the addition of tamoxifen to PF significantly enhances disease free survival of patients with primary breast cancer and positive nodes. The benefit, however, is limited to women 50 years of age or older and is associated with the ER and PgR content of their tumors. Aside from yielding no benefit to those women under the age of 50 with positive receptors, the addition of T to PF actually caused a significantly lower disease free survival in patients in this same age group whose tumors were receptor negative.

It is not clear why younger receptor negative patients should experience a lower survival with the addition of tamoxifen. Possibly the tamoxifen causes a change in the metabolism of PF either in the liver or at the level of the cancer cell. Whatever the explanation, this study clearly delineates the need to stratify patients according to prognostic factors, including receptor data, as subsets of breast cancer patients respond differently to adjuvant therapy.

Conclusion

Once the disease has become metastatic, the prognosis of patients with breast cancer is rarely in doubt. The past decade has been one of great progress in unraveling the mysteries of hormone dependent breast cancer. That steroid hormones are inextricably linked to the genesis and progression of breast cancer in undeniable. It is only through a more basic understanding of the mechanism of hormone modulation of breast cancer that we can fashion reasonable treatments for those patients with breast cancer.

REFERENCES

Adams D J, Edwards D P, McGuire W L 1983 Estrogen regulation of specific proteins as a mode of hormone action in breast cancer. In: Nowotny A (ed) Biomembranes, Plenum Press, New York, p 389–414

Allegra J C, Lippman M E 1980 Estrogen receptor status and the disease free interval in breast cancer. Recent Results in Cancer Research 71: 20–25

Antoniades K E, Spector H 1979 Correlation of estrogen receptor levels with histology and cytomorphology in human mammary cancer. American Journal of Clinical Pathology 71: 497–503

Beatson G T 1896 On the treatment of inoperable cases of carcinoma of the mamma: Suggestions for a new method of treatment, with illustrative cases. Lancet II: 104–107

Bertuzzi A, Daidone M F, DeFronzo G, Silverstini R 1981a Relationship among estrogen receptor, proliferative activity, and menopausal status in breast cancer. Breast Cancer Research and Treatment 1: 253–262

Bertuzzi A, Vezzoni P, Ronchi E 1981b Prognostic importance of progesterone receptors alone or in combination with estrogen receptors in node negative breast carcinoma. Proceedings of American Association of Clinical Research/American Society of Clinical Oncology 22:447

Bishop H M, Elston C W, Blamey R W, Haybittle S L, Nicholson R I, Griffiths K 1979 Relationship of oestrogen-receptor status to survival in breast cancer. Lancet 2: 283–284

Bloom H J G 1950 Prognosis in carcinoma of the breast. British Journal of Cancer 4: 259–288

Bloom W D, Tobin E H, Schreibman B, Degenshein G A 1980 The role of progesterone receptors in the management of advanced breast cancer. Cancer 45: 2992–2997

Brinkley D, Haybittle S L 1975 The curability of breast cancer. Lancet II: 95–97

Bronzert D A, Monaco M E, Pinkus L, Aitken S, Lippman M E 1981 Purification and properties of estrogen responsive thymidine kinase from human breast cancer. Cancer Research 41: 604–610

Bullock L P, Bardin C W, Sherman M R 1978 Androgenic, anti-andreogenic and synandrogenic action of progestins: Role of steric and allosteric interactions with androgen receptors. Endocrinology 103: 1768–1782

Campbell F C, Blamey R W, Elston C W, Nicholson R I, Griffiths K, Haybittle J L 1981 Oestrogen-receptor status and sites of metastasis in breast cancer. British Journal of Cancer 44: 456–459

Chamness G C, McGuire W L 1979 Methods for analyzing steroid receptors in human breast cancer. McGuire, W L (ed), Breast Cancer: Advances in Research and Treatment III. Plenum Press, New York, p 149–197

Chamness G C, McQuire W L 1982 Questions about histochemical methods for steroid receptors. Archives of Pathology and Laboratory Medicine 106: 53–54

Chamness G C, Mercer W D, McGuire W L 1980 Are histochemical methods for estrogen receptor valid? Journal of Histochemistry and Cytochemistry 28: 792–798

Champion H R, Wallace I W, Prescot R J 1972 Histology in breast cancer prognosis. British Journal of Cancer 26: 129–138

Clark G M, McGuire W L 1983 Progesterone receptors and human breast cancer. Breast Cancer Research and Treatment 3: 157–163

Clark G M, McGuire W L, Hubay C A, Pearson O H, Marshall J S 1983 Progesterone receptor as a prognostic factor in stage II breast cancer. New England Journal of Medicine 309: 1343–1347

Clemmensen J 1951 On the etiology of some human cancers. Journal of the National Cancer Institute 12: 1–21

Cole M P 1970 Prophylactic compared with therapeutic X-ray menopause. 2nd Tenovus Workshop on Breast Cancer 2–11

Cooke T, George W D, Griffiths K 1980 Possible tests for selection of adjuvant systemic therapy in early carcinoma of the breast. British Journal of Surgery 67: 747–750

Cutler S J, Devesa S S, Barclay T H C 1976 The magnitude of the breast cancer problem. Recent Results in Cancer Research 57: 1–9

Dao T L, Nemoto T, Chamberlain A, Bross I 1975 Adrenalectomy with radical mastectomy in the treatment of high risk breast cancer. Cancer 35: 478–482

Degenshein G A, Bloom N, Toben E 1980 The value of progesterone receptor assays in the management of advanced breast cancer. Cancer 46: 2789–2793

Delarue J C, May-Jevin F, Mouriesse H, Contesso G, Sancho-Gennier H 1981 Oestrogen and progesterone cytolosic receptors in clinically inflammatory tumors of the human breast. British Journal of Cancer 44: 911–916

deWaard F, Cornelius J P, Aoki K 1977 Breast cancer incidence according to weight and height in two cities of the Netherlands and in Aichi Prefecture, Japan. Cancer 49: 1269–1275

Drill V A 1981 An overview of studies on estrogens, oral contraceptives and breast cancer. Progress Drug Research 25: 159–187

Edwards D P, Adams D J, Savage W, McGuire W L 1980 Estrogen induced synthesis of specific proteins in human breast cancer cells. Biochemical and Biophysical Research Communications 93: 804–812

Edwards D P, Chamness G C, McGuire W L 1979 Estrogen and progesterone receptor proteins in breast cancer. Biochimica et Biophysica Acta 560: 457–486

Edwards D P, McGuire W L 1980 17α Estradiol is a biologically active estrogen in breast cancer cells in tissue culture. Endocrinology 107: 884–891

Edwards D P, Murthy S R, McGuire W L 1980 Effects of estrogen and anti-estrogen on DNA polymerase in human breast cancer. Cancer Research 40: 1722–1726

Feinleib M 1968 Breast Cancer and artificial menopause: A cohort study. Journal of the National Cancer Institute 41: 315–329

Fisher B, Redmond C, Brown A, Wickerman D L, Wolmack W, Allegra I, et al 1983a Influence of tumor estrogen and progesterone receptor levels on the response to tamoxifen and chemotherapy in primary breast cancer. Journal of Clinical Oncology 1: 227–241

Fisher B, Wickerham D L, Brown A, Redmond C K, with contributions by other NSABP Investigators 1983 Breast cancer estrogen and progesterone receptor values: their distribution, degree of concordance, and relation to number of positive axillary nodes. Journal of Clinical Oncology 1(6): 349–358

Fisher E R 1977 Pathology of breast cancer. In: McGuire W L (ed) Breast Cancer: Advances in Research and Treatment, Vol. 1, Plenum Press, New York, p 43–123

Fisher E R, Osborne C K, McGuire W L, Redmond C, Knight W A III, Fisher B et al 1981 Correlation of primary breast cancer histopathology and estrogen receptor content. Breast Cancer Research and Treatment 1: 37–41

Fisher E R, Redmond C K, Liu H, Rockette H, Fisher B, collaborating NSABP Investigators 1980 Correlation of estrogen receptor and pathologic characteristic of invasive breast cancer. Cancer 45: 349–353

Furmanski P, Saunders D E, Brooks S C, Rich M A and the Breast Cancer Prognostic Study Clinical and Pathology Associates 1980 The prognostic value of estrogen receptor determinations in patients with primary breast cancer. Cancer 46: 2794–2796

Gapinski P V, Donegan W I 1980 Estrogen receptors and breast cancer: prognostic and therapeutic implications. Surgery 88: 386–393

Gioanni J, Farges M F, Lalanne C M, Francoul M, Namer M 1979 Thymidine labeling index and estrogen receptor level in 64 human breast cancers. Biomedicine 31: 239–243

Hahnel R, Woodings T, Vivian A B 1979 Prognostic value of estrogen receptors in primary breast cancer. Cancer 44: 671–675

Hankin J H, Rawlings P H, Rawlings V 1978 Diet and breast cancer: a review. American Journal of Clinical Nutrition 31: 2005–2016

Hartveit F, Maartman-Moe H, Stou K F, Tangen M, Thorsen T 1980 Early recurrence in oestrogen receptor negative breast carcinomas. Acta Chirurgica Scandinavica 146: 93–95

Hartveit F, Thorenson S, Thorenson T, Tangen M 1981 Histologic grade and efferent vascular invasion in human breast cancer. British Journal of Cancer 44: 81–84

Horsley J S III, Horsley G W 1962 Twenty years of experience with prophylactic bilateral oophorectomy in the treatment of carcinoma of the breast. Annals of Surgery 155: 935–942

Horwitz K B, Costlow M E, McGuire W L 1975 MCF-7: A human breast cancer cell line with estrogen, androgen, progesterone and glucocorticoid receptor. Steroids 26: 785–795

Horwitz K B, McGuire W L 1978 Estrogen control of progesterone receptor in human breast cancer: correlation with nuclear processing of estrogen receptor. Journal of Biological Chemistry 253: 2223–2228

Horwitz K B, McGuire W L 1980 Studies on mechanisms of estrogen and antiestrogen action in human breast cancer. Recent Results in Cancer Research 71: 45–58

Horwitz K B, McGuire W L, Pearson O, Segaloff A 1975 Predicting response to endocrine therapy in human breast cancer: a hypothesis. Science 189: 726–727

Hubay C A, Pearson O H, Marshal J S, Stellato T A, Rhodes R S, DeBanne S M et al 1981 Adjuvant therapy of stage II breast cancer. Breast Cancer Research and Treatment 1: 77–82

Huggins C, Bergenstal D M 1951 Inhibition of human mammary and prostatic cancer by adrenalectomy. Cancer Research 12: 134–141

Huggins C, Dao T L 1954 Characteristics of adrenal dependent mammary cancer. Annals of Surgery 12: 497–501

Jungblut P W, Hughes A, Gaues J, Kallweit E, Maschler I, Parl F et al R K 1979 Mechanisms involved in the regulation of steroid receptor levels. Journal of Steroid Biochemistry 11: 273–278

Keifer W S, Scott J C 1975 A clinical appraisal of patients following long-term contraception. American Journal of Obstetrics and Gynecology 122: 446–457

Kelsey J L 1979 A review of the epidemiology of human breast cancer. Epidemiologic Reviews 1: 74–109

Kennedy B J, Mielke P W, Fortuny I E 1964 Therapeutic castration versus prophylactic castration in breast cancer. Surgery, Gynecology and Obstetrics 118: 524–540

Kinne D W, Ashikari R, Butler A, Menendez-Botet C, Rosen P R, Schwartz M 1981 Estrogen receptor protein in breast cancer as a predictor of recurrence. Cancer 47: 2364–2367

Knazek R, Lippman M E, Chopra H 1977 Formation of solid human mammary carcinoma in vitro. Journal of the National Cancer Institute 58: 419–435

Knight W A III, Livingston R B, Gregory E J, McGuire W L 1977 Estrogen receptor is an independent prognostic factor for early recurrence in breast cancer. Cancer Research 37: 4669–4671

Korenman S G 1980 Oestrogen window hypothesis of the aetiology of breast cancer. Lancet I: 700–701

Kute T E, Muss H B, Anderson D, Crumb K, Miller B, Burns D, Duke L 1981 Relationship of steroid receptors, cell kinetics, and clinical status in patients with breast cancer. Cancer Research 41: 3524–3529

Leake R E, Laing L, McArdle C, Smith D C 1981 Soluble and nuclear oestrogen receptor status in human breast cancer in relation to prognosis. British Journal of Cancer 43: 67–71

Lilienfield A M 1956 Relationship of cancer of the female breast to artificial menopause and marital status. Cancer 9: 927–934

Lilienfield A M, Coombs J, Bross I D J, Chamberlain A 1975 Marital and reproductive experience in a community-wide epidemiologic study of breast cancer. Johns Hopkins Medical Journal 136: 157–162

Lippman M E 1981 Hormonal regulation of human breast cancer cells in vitro. In: Pike M C, Siiteri P K, Welsch C W (eds) Banbury Report 8: Hormones and Breast Cancer. Cold Spring Harbour Laboratory.

Lippman M E, Aitken S C 1980 Estrogen and antiestrogen effects on thymidine utilization by MCF-7 human cancer cells in tissue culture. Progress in Cancer Research and Therapy 14: 3–19

Lippman M E, Bolan G 1975 Oestrogen-responsive human breast cancer in long term tissue culture. Nature 256: 592–595

Logan W P D 1953 Marriage and childbearing in relation to cancer of the breast and uterus. Lancet II: 1199–1202

MacMahon B, Cole P, Brown J 1973 Etiology of human breast cancer: a review. Journal of National Cancer Institute 50: 21–42

MacMahon B, Cole P, Lin T M, Lowe C R, Mina A P, Ravnihan B, Salber E J, Valaoras G, Yvasa S 1970 Age at first birth and breast cancer risk. Bulletin of the World Health Organization 43: 209–221

MacMohan B, Trichopsulos D, Brown J, Andersen A P, Aoki K, Cole P et al 1982 Age at menarche, probability of ovulation and breast cancer. International Journal of Cancer 29: 13–16

Martin P M, Rolland P H, Jacquemier J, Rolland A M, Toye M 1979 Multiple steroid receptors in human breast cancer. III. Relationship between steroid receptors and the state of differentiation and the activity of carcinomas throughout the pathologic features. Cancer Chemotherapy and Pharmacology 2: 115–120

Maynard P V, Davies C J, Blamey R W, Elston C W, Johnson J, Griffiths K 1978 Relationship between oestrogen-receptor content and histologic grade in human primary breast tumors. British Journal of Cancer 38: 745–748

McCarty K S, Barton T K, Fetter B F, Woodard B H, Mossler J A, Reeves W et al 1980 Correlation of estrogen and progesterone receptors with histologic differentiation in mammary carcinoma. Cancer 46: 2851–2858

McGuire W L, Carbone P P, Sears M E, Eocher G C 1975 Estrogen receptors in human breast cancer: an overview. In: McGuire W L, Vollmer E P, Carbone P P (eds) Estrogen Receptors in Human Breast Cancer, Raven Press, New York, p 1–7

McGuire W L, Horwitz K B 1978 Progesterone receptors in breast cancer. In: McGuire W L (ed) Hormones Receptors and Breast Cancer, Raven Press, New York p 31–42

Meakin J W, Allt W E C, Beale F A, Brown T C, Bush R S, Clark R M et al 1979 Ovarian irradiation and prednisone therapy following surgery and radiotherapy for carcinoma of the breast. Canadian Medical Association Journal 120: 1221–1229

Meyer J R, Rao B R, Stevens S C, White W L 1977 Low incidence of estrogen receptor in breast carcinomas with rapid rates of cellular replication. Cancer 40: 2290–2298

Millis R R 1980 Correlation of hormone receptors with pathologic features in human breast cancer. Cancer 46: 2869–2871

Muss H B, Kute T R, Cooper M R, Marshall R C 1980 The correlation of estrogen and progesterone receptors with DNA histograms in patients with advanced breast cancer. Proceedings of the American Association of Cancer Research/American Society of Clinical Oncology 21:172

Nevinny H B, Nevinny D, Rosoff C B, Hall T C, Muench H 1969 Prophylactic oophorectomy in breast cancer therapy. American Journal of Surgery 117: 531–535

Nissen Meyer R 1964 Prophylactic endocrine treatment in carcinomas of the breast. Clinical Radiology 15: 152–160

Norris H J, Taylor H B 1965 Prognosis of mucinous (gelatinous) carcinoma of the breast. Cancer 18: 879–885

Osborne C K, McGuire W L 1983 Endocrine therapy of metastatic breast cancer. In: Krieger D T, Bardin C W (eds) Current Therapy in Endocrinology, B C Decker Inc, Toronto, p 334–341

Osborne C K, Yochmowitz M D, Knight W A III, McGuire W L 1980 The value of estrogen and progesterone receptors in the treatment of breast cancer. Cancer 46: 2884–2888

Paffenbarger R S Jr, Fasil E, Simmons M E, Kampert J B 1977 Cancer risk as related to use of oral contraceptives during fertile years. Cancer 39: 1887–1891

Palshoff T: Adjuvant endocrine therapy 1981 Canadian Journal of Surgery 24: 379–384

Panko W B, McLeod R M 1978 Unchanged nuclear receptors for estrogen in breast. Cancer Research 38: 1948–1951

Pinchon M F, Pallud C, Brunet M, Milgrom E 1980 Relationship of presence of progesterone receptors to prognosis in early breast cancer. Cancer Research 40: 3357–3360

Ramazzini B 1713 Diseases of workers. Translated by W C Wright 1964, Hafner Publishing Co, New York, p 167–202

Ravdin R G, Lewison E F, Slack W H, Dao T L, Garcher B, State D, Fisher B 1970 Results of a clinical trial concerning the worth of prophylactic oophorectomy for breast carcinoma. Surgery, Gynecology and Obstetrics 131: 1055–1061

Riberio G, Pamer M K 1983 Adjuvant tamoxifen for operable carcinoma of the breast: report of a clinical trial by the Christie Hospital and Holt Radium Institute. British Medical Journal 286: 827–830

Rich M A, Funnenski P, Brooks S C and the Breast Cancer Prognostic Study Surgery and Pathology Associates 1978 Prognostic value of estrogen receptor determinations in patients with breast cancer. Cancer Research 38: 4296–4298

Rochefort H, Borgna J L 1981 Differences between oestrogen receptor activation by oestrogen and antioestrogen. Nature 292: 257–259

Rolland P H, Jacquemier J, Martin P U 1980 Histologic differentation in human breast cancer is related to steroid receptors and stromal elastosis. Cancer Chemotherapy and Pharmacology 5: 73–77

Russo J, Soule H D, McGrath C, Rich M A 1976 Reexpression of the original tumor pattern by a human breast carcinoma cell line (MCF-7) in sponge culture. Journal of the National Cancer Institute 56: 279–283

Saez S, Chouret C, Majer M, Chix F 1981 Estradiol and progesterone receptor as prognostic factors in human primary breast tumors. Proceedings of American Association of Clinical Oncology/American Society of Clinical Oncology 21:139

Samaan W A, Buydar A U, Aldinger K A, Schultz P N, Yong K P, Romsdahl M M, Martin R 1981 Estrogen receptor: a prognostic factor in breast cancer. Cancer 47: 554–560

Schinzinger A 1889 Über Carcinoma Mammae. Verhandlungen der Gesellschaft Fuer Orthopaedische Chirurgie 18:28

Sherman B M, Korenman S G 1974 Inadequate corpus luteum function: pathophysiological interpretation of human breast cancer epidemiology. Cancer 33: 1306–1312

Sherman B M, Korenman G, Wallace R B 1982 Corpus luteum dysfunction and the epidemiology of breast cancer: a reconsideration. Breast Cancer Research and Treatment 1: 287–296

Shinghakowinata A, Potter H G, Buroker T R, Samals S, Brooks S C, Vaitkevicius V 1976 Estrogen receptor and the natural course of breast cancer. Annals of Surgery 183: 77–84

Silfversward C, Gustaf'sson J, Gustaf'sson S A, Humla S, Nordenskjold B, Wallgren A, Wrange O 1980 Estrogen receptor concentrations in 269 cases of histologically classified human breast cancer. Cancer 45: 2001–2005

Soule H D, Vasquez J, Ling A, Albert S, Brennan M 1973 A human cell line from a pleural effusion derived from a breast carcinoma. Journal of the National Cancer Institute 51: 1409–1414

Stewart J F, King R J B, Sexton S A, Millis R R, Ruben R D, Hayward J L 1981 Oestrogen receptors, sites of metastatic disease and survival in recurrent breast cancer. European Journal of Cancer 17: 449–453

Taylor G W 1939 Ovarian sterilisation for breast cancer. Surgery, Gynecology and Obstetrics 68:452

Taylor H B, Norris H J 1970 Well-differentiated carcinoma of the breast. Cancer 25: 687–692

Thomas D B 1982 Noncontraceptive exogenous estrogens and risk of breast cancer: a review. Breast Cancer Research and Treatment 2: 203–211

Trichopolous D, MacMahon B, Cole P 1972 Menopause and breast cancer risk. Journal of the National Cancer Institute 48: 605–613

Vessey M, Doll R, Reto R 1976 Along term followup study of women using different methods of contraception. Journal of Biosocial Science 8: 373–427

Vessey M, Doll R, Sutton P M 1972 Oral contraceptives and breast neoplasia: a retrospective study. British Medical Journal 3: 719–724

Walt A J, Shinghakowinata A, Brooks S C, Cortez A 1976 The surgical implications of the estrophile protein estimations in carcinoma of the breast. Surgery 80: 506–512

Young P C M, Ehrlich C E, Einhorn L H 1980 Relationship between steroid receptors and response to endocrine therapy and cytotoxic chemotherapy in metastatic breast cancer. Cancer 46: 2961–2963

Zava D T, Chamness G C, Horwitz K B, McGuire W L 1977 Biologically active estrogen receptor in the absence of estrogen. Science 196: 663–664

Zava D T, McGuire W L 1978 Human Breast Cancer: Androgen action mediated by estrogen receptor. Science 199: 787–788

Zumoff B, Fishman J, Bradlow H L, Hellman S 1975 Hormone profiles in hormone dependent cancer. Cancer Research 35: 3365–3373

4 Breast pain: clinical spectrum and practical management

ROBERT MANSEL

Pain in the breast is the single most common reason for which patients seek medical advice about their breasts, both in general practice and in the surgical clinic. The scant attention breast pain receives in either general, or specialist texts devoted to breast diseases, highlights the generally poor understanding of the aetiology, classification and management of this symptom.

Despite popular opinion, neuroticism is not a major aetiological factor, and pain as the sole presenting symptom is not a common feature of operable breast cancer. There are 3 main groups of breast pain (Table 4.1). The occurrence, aetiology and management of the physiological causes of breast pain are well documented and will not be discussed further as they are generally self-limiting conditions. Pain due to an identifiable primary condition, forms the second group, which is also summarized in Table 4.1. This group is not discussed in detail as the management is that of the primary condition. However, the management of non-cyclical pain due to plasma cell mastitis is discussed in the section on treatment. The third (and largest) group is that of breast pain without a well defined primary cause and which may occur in a localised or diffuse distribution and may or may not be associated with nodularity. This group may be thought of as an idiopathic group and is conveniently described by the term mastalgia. There are two principal patterns of mastalgia, cyclical and non-cyclical, and these will be discussed in detail in this chapter, placing these in perspective against the other causes of breast pain with which they may be confused and outlining a practical plan of management.

Incidence

The exact incidence of mastalgia is unknown but it is certainly common and varies from 1–2 days of premenstrual aching, which most women would regard as normal, up to 3–4 weeks of severe pain each cycle. Haagensen has estimated that 16% of all women during their lifetime will seek surgical advice for abnormal physiology or benign lesions of physiological origin

48

Table 4.1 Causes of breast pain

Physiological
  Telarche
  Gynaecomastia
  Pregnancy
Secondary to an identifiable primary condition
  Infection
    — Bacterial/Viral (Bornholm's disease)
  Trauma
    — Fat necrosis/haematoma
    — Mondor's disease
    — Post-biopsy
  Plasma cell mastitis
  Cancer
  Drug induced gynaecomastia
  Referred pain
    — Gallstones/lung disease
    — Tietze's disease (painful costochondral syndrome)
  Exogenous oestrogen administration
Breast pain with no obvious physical or pathological basis
  Cyclical Mastalgia
  Non-cyclical Mastalgia

(Haagensen, 1971). Breast pain has been shown to be the commonest reason for consultation on breast problems in general practice (Nichols et al, 1980).

Classification

A sensible classification of mastalgia has been prevented by the widespread confusion of clinical terms used to describe benign breast disease (BBD), such as chronic mastitis or mastopathy; with pathological terms, such as fibroadenosis or cystic disease. These terms have neither clinical nor pathological precision and certainly do not describe mastalgia which is obviously a symptom. Geschickter (1945) used the term mastodynia to describe pain with accompanying breast nodularity and this term is still used in Europe today, although with a less precise definition. The term mastalgia is used in this text to mean simply breast pain which may exist by itself or in conjunction with diffuse nodularity of the breast.

A special study was set up within the Cardiff Breast Clinic in 1973 with the aim of producing a clinically-based classification of mastalgia. After exclusion of cancer by clinical examination and mammography, a careful history of the pain and its related features and a relevant endocrine and menstrual history was recorded (Preece et al 1976). To date a total of 600 patients have been classified and several patterns of pain have emerged (Table 4.1).

The major pattern is the cyclical pronounced pattern, which as its name suggests, is related to the menstrual cycle and hence is seen only in pre-menopausal women. Typically it occurs in women of mean age 34 yrs (range 16–50), is described as a tenderness or heaviness in the outer half of the breast and is frequently accompanied by nodularity. In severe cases the pain begins soon after menstruation and continues until it is relieved by the next menstru-

Daily Breast Pain Chart

Name

Record the amount of breast pain you experience each day by shading in each box as illustrated.

■ Severe pain

◪ Mild pain

⦿ No pain

For example:- If you get severe breast pain on the fifth of the month then shade in completely the square under 5. Please note the day your period starts each month with the letter 'P'.

Please bring this card with you on each visit.

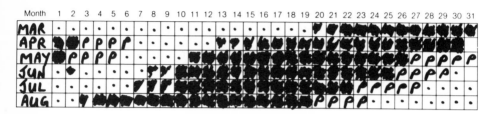

Fig. 4.1 Breast pain chart showing the cyclical pattern of mastalgia.

ation, although most patients begin to have symptoms around mid cycle i.e. during the luteal phase of the cycle (Fig. 4.1).

The second commonest pattern has no temporal relationship to the menstrual cycle and is designated non-cyclical. It occurs in both pre and post menopausal patients and is usually described as having a 'burning' or 'drawing' quality. Nodularity is uncommon and, in contrast to the cyclical pattern, the medial half or subareolar region of the breast is mainly affected. Clinically, this pattern can be separated from the cyclical by using a simple pain chart which records the relationship of the symptoms to the menstrual cycle (Fig. 4.2).

Tietze's syndrome was found to be the third largest group presenting to the Mastalgia Clinic and has been well known since the first description of the painful costo-chondral junctions by Tietze in 1921. It is a chronic pain which is distinguished from the non-cyclical pattern by the characteristic tenderness of the rib cartilages deep to medial half of the breast. This condition should be classified as a referred, rather than a true, breast pain (Table 4.1).

A fourth and smaller group is the post trauma pattern which occurs in a breast biopsy scar either immediately post-biopsy or some time later. This well localised pain is found more commonly following a wound complication such as infection or haematoma. These four groups account for most cases of breast pain referred to the surgeon but it should be noted that many conditions in the lungs, upper abdomen or thoracic spine may be responsible for referred pain in the breast.

Breast pain as the sole presenting symptom of breast cancer occurs in less than 10% of operable breast cancer (Preece et al, 1982), and further, presents no unique features that would help in diagnosis. The classification presented above is based on symptoms and does not correlate with any specific histological changes found in the breast. Despite this apparent drawback, the classification does have practical clinical value as will be seen later.

Daily Breast Pain Chart

Name

Record the amount of breast pain you experience each day by shading in each box as illustrated.

■ **Severe pain**

◪ **Mild pain**

● **No pain**

For example:- If you get severe breast pain on the fifth of the month then shade in completely the square under 5. Please note the day your period starts each month with the letter 'P'.

Please bring this card with you on each visit.

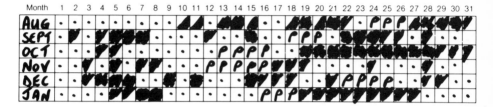

Fig. 4.2 Breast pain chart showing the non-cyclical pattern of mastalgia.

Aetiology of Mastalgia

There are three principal theories of the causes of mastalgia: neuroticism, oedema due to water retention and hormonal imbalance. Early evidence supporting these theories was largely anecdotal but the advent of accurate hormone estimation by radio-immunoassay has enabled proper scientific examination of these hypotheses.

The theory of neuroticism was based on impressions rather than hard facts (Cooper, 1829) but these views are still prevalent today. However, a study comparing the neurotic traits of mastalgia patients with other surgical outpatients and normals showed conclusively that mastalgia patients were no more neurotic than other surgical outpatients (Preece et al, 1978).

The supporters of the theory of water retention pointed to the documented breast swelling occurring in the luteal phase of the cycle (Milligan et al, 1975) and the apparent beneficial effects of diuretics in mastalgia. Again, scientific study fails to support these contentions. In a study measuring total body water by isotopic methods, there was no difference in the mean water gain between the 5th and 25th days of the cycle when symptomless controls were compared with mastalgia patients (Preece et al, 1975). Reports of the efficacy of diuretics are anecdotal and are almost certainly due to placebo effects, but despite this weight of evidence, diuretics remain the commonest therapy prescribed for mastalgia by the general practitioner.

An hormonal abnormality thus appears to be the most likely theory for the aetiology of mastalgia but hard scientific evidence is lacking for most of the proposed abnormalities. Early workers proposed ovarian hypersecretion but were not able to measure the hormones directly (Atkins, 1940; Geschickter, 1945). After progesterone and oestrogen were identified and measured directly

in serum, it was suggested that the primary problem was either a pure hypersecretion of oestradiol or a deficiency in progesterone leading to a relative hyper-
oestrogenism. Mauvais-Jarvis and his colleagues in Paris reported a clear
deficiency of luteal phase progesterone in their 'mastodynia' patients (Sitruk-
Ware et al, 1977) and seemed to prove the theory of luteal insufficiency.
However a careful longitudinal study in Britain failed to show any progesterone
deficiency (England et al, 1981) and a 24 hour sampling study of American
patients also failed to support the luteal insufficiency theory (Malarkey et al,
1977a) A more recent study of salivary progesterone levels throughout the
menstrual cycle in patients with benign breast disease has also failed to detect
low luteal progesterone levels (Read et al, 1985). The theory of luteal insufficiency thus remains unproven.

The discovery of human prolactin as a separate entity about a decade ago,
raised the possibility of increased breast stimulation secondary to hyperprolactinaemia as a possible aetiology. Measurement of plasma prolactin is made
difficult by the pulsatile secretion and diurnal variation of the hormone and
early studies showed no difference between breast disease cases and normal
controls. A study of daily basal blood prolactin estimations did show a small,
but statistically significant, elevation in women with cystic disease but all read-
ings remained within the normal range (Cole et al, 1977). A 24 hour profile
of prolactin secretion showed no differences between benign breast disease
patients and controls by day or night. (Malarkey et al 1977b). These studies
suggested that there was no overt hyperprolactinaemia in mastalgia patients.
The fact that breast symptoms are relatively uncommon in patients with
hyperprolactinaemia secondary to pituitary adenomas, is further circumstantial
evidence of a lack of a major role for prolactin in the aetiology of mastalgia.
However, recent studies of thyrotrophin releasing hormone (TRH)-stimulated
levels of prolactin have shown some interesting results. Peters et al (1981)
demonstrated an increased peak secretion of prolactin in their breast pain
(mastodynia) group when compared with controls. These findings have
recently been confirmed in a study where both TRH-stimulated and domperidone stimulated prolactin secretion was shown to be significantly increased in
patients with cyclical mastalgia compared with normal controls and women
with non-cyclical mastalgia (Kumar et al, 1984). This latter study also showed
that thyroid function was identical in the mastalgia and control groups, unlike
the German study where mild hypothyroidism was also found (Peters et al,
1981). These results certainly suggest a central endocrine defect in cyclical
mastalgia but so far no similar abnormality has been demonstrated in the non-
cyclical group.

There are several other general aetiological theories of BBD, which relate
to dietary factors. Minton has suggested that a high intake of methylxanthines
in the form of caffeine or cola is a risk factor for the genesis of BBD in the
USA but this factor seems less important in other countries, probably due to
the lower intake of caffeine (Minton, 1981).

A more recent hypothesis is that essential fatty acid intake is suboptimal in
the 'Western' diet and this leads to interference with prostaglandin metabolism

which results in amplification of prolactin stimulation of the breast (Horrobin, 1979). This hypothesis awaits confirmation by further work.

To summarise the current knowledge on the aetiology, it can be said that a gross endocrine defect is unlikely in mastalgia but a subtle abnormality of the control of prolactin or some other hormone appears more likely.

Management of Mastalgia

The most important step in managing mastalgia is to exclude breast cancer by careful clinical examination and mammography where indicated. As has been noted, mastalgia as the sole presenting feature of cancer is uncommon, especially in the cyclical patients who have a mean age of around 33 years. Once the clinician is sure that cancer is not the cause of the presenting mastalgia, this fact should be communicated to the patient, as most patients with mastalgia consult the doctor in order to be reassured that they do not have cancer. Adequate reassurance is all that is required for the majority of patients (85% in the Cardiff Breast Clinic) and this is successful because of the removal of fear of cancer. Symptoms are obviously not directly affected by reassurance but rather the patient's attitude to her symptoms.

However, some 15% of mastalgia patients suffer pain of sufficient intensity to interfere with daily activities such as housework or looking after children. Even more important is the irritability produced by prolonged sore breasts, in both the patient and her marital partner. It is these patients who return to the clinic with continued complaints of mastalgia and are regarded as neurotic by many surgeons who feel unable or unwilling to help the problem of persistent mastalgia.

General Measures

Some simple advice is worth considering at the outset. A detailed history should be taken in order to separate out the physiological and secondary causes of mastalgia such as exogenous oestrogen administration, prolactinomas or infections of the breast. Next, causes of referred breast pain such as gallstones, lung disease or herpes zoster should be excluded.

Geschickter (1945) stated simply that the treatment should 'exclude cancer, rule out infection and give support', and many women find that a well-fitted brassiere seems to help and may need to be worn at night for maximum effect. Brassieres specially fitted in the breast clinic have been reported to be helpful (Wilson & Sellwood, 1976), although they are unlikely to help the most severe cases. Diuretics are often advocated but there are no controlled studies supporting their use and mastalgia patients do not specifically retain water as noted above.

At this point, the pattern of mastalgia should be determined and although this can be done in some cases by taking a careful history, it is more convenient to ask the patient to record the timing of her symptoms on a simple pain chart such as illustrated in Figure 4.1.

For practical purposes this will split the patients into the cyclical and non-cyclical pattern, the latter including Tietze's cases which are indistinguishable from the non-cyclical pattern on pain charts but are separated by the finding of tender, swollen costo-chondral junctions.

The distinction between cyclical and non-cyclical patterns is important, as it appears that the cyclical patients may selectively respond to hormonal therapy as noted in the following section.

Drug Therapy

The drug therapies for mastalgia are generally directed towards correction of each of the principal hypotheses of aetiology and are perhaps less empirical than older treatments (Table 4.2). Reports of treatment for mastalgia must however be examined critically as the condition is a symptom, with few objective signs and as such, any treatment will have placebo effects which must be controlled. Unfortunately, most studies of therapy for mastalgia have been uncontrolled and have made no allowance for the placebo effect.

Table 4.2 Mastalgia: Aetiological hypotheses and treatments

Hyperoestrogenism	Androgens/anti-oestrogens (Tamoxifen)
Luteal insufficiency	Progesterone/Progestogens
Hyperprolactinaemia	Bromocriptine (dopamine agonist)
Increased gonadotrophin	Danazol (antigonadotrophin)
Dietary methylxanthines	Caffeine restriction
Dietary essential fatty acids (EFA)	Evening primrose oil (EFA supplement)
Miscellaneous	Pyridoxine/thyroid hormones/Vitamin B_1.

In 1940 Atkins showed that testosterone was effective in reducing the mastalgia associated with 'chronic mastitis', but found that the androgenic side effects were unacceptable (Atkins, 1940). The anti-oestrogen tamoxifen has also been used to treat mastalgia symptoms in an open study (Ricciardi & Ianni-ruberto, 1979) but the drug has not officially been approved for this indication in most countries, and suffers from the theoretical disadvantage of inducing a rise in serum oestradiol in premenopausal women.

Correction of alleged luteal insufficiency by exogenous progestogens has been used by Mauvais-Jarvis and his group using oral administration of lynes-trenol combined with skin creams containing progestogen in uncontrolled studies. (Mauvais-Jarvis et al, 1979). One controlled study using lynestrenol 10 mg on days 10–24 of the cycle showed a significant advantage to the progestogen but the improvement was mainly in thermographic appearances, which are highly subjective and show little correlation with mastalgia (Colin et al, 1978).

The value of progestogens for mastalgia thus remains an open question, but a double blind trial of dydrogesterone against placebo in the premenstrual tension syndrome failed to show any advantage for progestogen administration in the control of breast pain although the other premenstrual symptoms improved. (Day, 1979).

Precise manipulation of prolactin levels became possible with the discovery of the dopamine agonist, bromocriptine, and early uncontrolled reports suggested that the drug was effective in mastalgia. A controlled trial in premenstrual tension patients showed that the breast symptoms of this syndrome were relieved by bromocriptine (Benedek-Jaszmann & Hearn-Sturtevant, 1976). The value of bromocriptine in cyclical mastalgia was confirmed in a large, double blind, placebo-controlled trial using a dose of 2.5 mg b.d. (Mansel et al, 1978). This trial also showed that patients with a non-cyclical pattern failed to respond to prolactin lowering therapy. Further controlled trials have confirmed the efficacy of bromocriptine, in mastalgia (Montgomery et al, 1979; Blichert-Toft et al, 1979; Durning & Sellwood, 1982). Side effects are common on bromocriptine, especially nausea and dizziness which may affect 30–40% of patients, although they can be reduced considerably by increasing the drug slowly in 1.25 mg increments. Bromocriptine appears to be effective despite the fact that patients with mastalgia have basal prolactin levels within the normal range.

Another agent, danazol, was initially introduced for the treatment of endometriosis but Greenblatt suggested that its antigonadotrophic action might be useful in damping down the symptoms of BBD (Greenblatt et al 1971). A number of papers followed from the same group and others, reporting improvement in symptoms and resolution of nodules in mastalgia but all of these studies were conducted on an open basis (Lauerson & Wilson, 1976; Asch & Greenblatt, 1977; Greenblatt et al, 1980). A double blind, placebo controlled study has however confirmed the efficacy of danazol in reducing pain and nodularity in cyclical mastalgia patients using a dose of 200–400 mg daily which is lower than that used in endometriosis (Mansel et al, 1982). Danazol appears to work by inhibiting ovulation as patients on the drug in this latter trial were shown to have very low luteal progesterone values, but a local effect cannot be discounted as danazol has been shown to bind to hormone receptors on human breast cancer cells. Side effects are also fairly common and are mainly due to the weak androgenic effect of danazol which gives rise to acne, weight gain and amenorrhoea, all of which are disliked by women. More recently, doses as low as 100 mg daily are being used and are effective with dramatically reduced side effects. Amenorrhoea will occur in 50% of women at 400 mg daily but occurs rarely at a dose of 100 mg daily.

The remaining treatments are still under evaluation or are unproven. Caffeine withdrawal has been shown to be useful in patients drinking a large amount of coffee (Minton et al, 1979) but may not be applicable in all countries. Claims of the value of pyridoxine, vitamin B_1, vitamin E and thyroid hormones are based on uncontrolled studies and have not been independently confirmed (Estes, 1981; Renwick, 1979; London et al, 1982). The supplementation of the diet by EFA's in the form of evening primrose oil is currently undergoing evaluation in controlled trials and has the potential advantage that the treatment has virtually no side effects.

Treatment of non-cyclical pain
Drug therapy is generally less effective for non-cyclical pain than for cyclical pain and a controlled trial showed little effect of a hormonal treatment in the former group when patients were stratified into the 2 patterns of pain (Mansel

et al, 1978). In the Cardiff Mastalgia Clinic an overall response of 40% was obtained using either bromocriptine or danazol for non-cyclical pain. This response rate is only marginally better than the placebo rate in non-cyclical pain. As in cyclical pain, reassurance of the absence of cancer is important especially in this group who have a mean age of 43 years. Patients with Tietze's syndrome have a non-cyclical pain pattern, but are distinguished by the presence of tender costal junctions anteriorly. These patients often respond to a local injection of lignocaine and hydrocortisone infiltrated around the painful cartilage.

When non-cyclical pain is found to be localised to a small area in the breast on several different consultations, it may respond to local injection of local anaesthetic and depot steroid (Crile, 1977). Local excision of a painful area cures the pain in 50% of the cases but excision is of no value in cases with diffuse pain. Surgery may also be helpful in cases of non-cylical mastalgia due to subareolar plasma cell mastitis, where a major duct excision may cure the mastalgia and concomittant nipple discharge (Urban, 1963). Recent work has also shown that the inflammation and nipple discharge of plasma cell mastitis may also respond to bromocriptine therapy (Peters et al, 1982).

Role of Surgery
With the exception of the localised excisions detailed above for non-cyclical mastalgia, surgery has little to offer in most cases of diffuse mastalgia. Subcutaneous mastectomy is sometimes performed for severe intractable mastalgia but even this radical procedure may fail to control the pain. In the Cardiff Breast Clinic, during the last 5 years when 300 cases of mastalgia have been treated by drugs, only 3 subcutaneous mastectomies have been performed, thus demonstrating the infrequency of this procedure for the treatment of mastalgia. Patients being considered for the radical procedure of subcutaneous mastectomy should always be referred for a prior psychiatric opinion.

The Natural History of Mastalgia

Despite the large amount of literature published on the subsequent cancer risk of a history of BBD, little has been written on the natural history of breast symptoms. Geschickter (1945) noted that spontaneous resolution of mastodynia does occur in a number of cases. A detailed follow up of the cyclical and non-cyclical groups in the Cardiff Mastalgia Clinic showed that 65% still had pain after a follow up ranging from 2–7 years. (Wisbey et al, 1983). In addition, spontaneous relief in the cyclical group was generally related to an hormonal event such as the menopause or pregnancy while relief in the non-cyclical group was not related to an hormonal event— a further point of difference between the two patterns. It was clear that patients who first experience severe mastalgia in their second decade are likely to suffer recurring symptoms over many years. The implication is that the young patient with severe mastalgia is likely to require therapy over many years and it is our practice to treat in short courses of 4–6 months, in order to limit possible long-term suppression of the pituitary-ovarian axis and to allow detection of spontaneous resolution of symptoms. In the cyclical group, at least the onset of the menopause will predictably cure their symptoms.

REFERENCES

Asch R H, Greenblatt R B 1977 The use of an impeded androgen-danzol-in the management of benign breast disorders. American Journal of Obstetrics and Gynaecology 127: 130–134

Atkins H J B, 1940 Treatment of chronic mastitis. Lancet II: 411–413

Benedek-Jaszmann L J, Hearn-Sturtevant M D 1976 Premenstrual tension and functional infertility Lancet I: 1095–1098

Blichert-Toft M, Anderson A N, Henriksen O B, Mygind T 1979 Treatment of mastalgia with bromocriptine: a double blind crossover study. British Medical Journal 1:237

Cooper A, 1829 Illustrations of the diseases of the breast Part I Longman, Rees, Orme, Brown and Green, London

Colin C, Gaspard U, Lambotte R 1978 Relationship of mastodynia with its endocrine environment and treatment in a double blind trial with lynestrenol. Archives of Gynecology (Munchen) 225: 7–13

Cole E N, Sellwood R A, England P C, Griffiths K 1977 Serum prolactin concentrations in benign breast disease throughout the menstrual cycle. European Journal of Cancer 13: 597–603

Crile G Jr 1977 Injection of steroids in painful breasts. American Journal of Surgery 133: 705

Day J B 1979 Clinical trials in the premenstrual syndrome. Current Medical Research and Opinion (Suppl 5): 40–45

Durning P, Sellwood R A 1982 Bromocriptine in severe cyclical breast pain. British Journal of Surgery 69: 248–249

England P C, Sellwood R A, Knyba R E, Irvine J D B 1981 Serum androgen levels and the menstrual cycle in women with benign or malignant breast disease. Clinical Oncology 7: 213–219

Estes N C 1981 Mastodynia due to fibrocystic disease of the breast controlled with thyroid hormone. American Journal of Surgery 142: 764–766

Geschickter C F 1945 Diseases of the breast 2nd edn. Lippincott, Philadelphia Ch 8

Greenblatt R B, Dmowski W P, Mahesh V B, Scholer H F L 1971 Clinical studies with an antigonadotropin—danazol. Fertility and Sterility 22: 102–112

Greenblatt R B, Nezhat C, Ben-Nun I 1980 The treatment of benign breast disease with danazol. Fertility and Sterility 34: 242–245

Haagensen C D 1971 Diseases of the breast, 2nd edn. revised, Saunders, Philadelphia Ch 4, p 101

Horrobin D F 1979 Cellular basis of prolactin action: involvement of cyclic nucleotides polyamines, prostaglandins, steroids, thyroid hormones, Na/K ATPases and calcium; relevance to breast cancer and the menstrual cycle. Medical Hypotheses 5: 599–614

Kumar S, Mansel R E, Hughes L E, Woodhead J S, Edwards C A, Scanlon M F, Newcombe R G 1984 Prolactin response to TRH stimulation and dopaminergic inhibition in benign breast disease. Cancer 53: 1311–15

Lauerson N H, Wilson K H 1976 The effect of danazol in the treatment of chronic cystic mastitis. Obstetrics and Gynaecology 48: 93–98

London R S, Sundarman G S, Goldstein P J 1982 Medical management of mammary dysplasia Obstetrics and Gynaecology 59: 519–523

Malarkey W B, Schroeder L L, Stevens V C, James A G, Lanese R R, 1977a, Twenty-four-hour pre-operative endocrine profiles in women with benign and malignant breast disease. Cancer Research 37: 4655–4659

Malarkey W B, Schroeder L L, Stevens V C, James A G, Lanese R R, 1977b Disordered nocturnal prolactin regulation in women with breast cancer. Cancer Research 37: 4650–4654

Mansel R E, Wisbey J R, Hughes L E 1982 Controlled trial of the antigonadotropin danazol in painful nodular benign breast disease. Lancet I: 928–931

Mansel R E, Preece P E, Hughes L E 1978 A double blind trial of the prolactin inhibitor Bromocriptine in painful benign breast disease. British Journal of Surgery 65: 724–727

Mauvais-Jarvis P, Sitruk-Ware R, Kuttenn F, Sterkers N 1979 Luteal phase insufficiency: a common pathophysiologic factor in development of benign and malignant breast disease. In:

Bulbrook R D, Taylor D J (eds) Commentaries on Research in Breast Disease. Alan R Liss Inc., New York 1: 25–29

Milligan D, Drife J D, Short R V 1975 Changes in breast volume during normal menstrual cycle and after oral contraceptives. British Medical Journal 4: 494–496

Minton J P, Foecking M K, Webster D J T, Mathews R H 1979 Response of fibrocystic disease to caffeine withdrawal and correlation of cyclic nucleotides with breast disease. American Journal of Obstetrics and Gynaecology 135: 157–158

Minton J P, Abou-Issa H, Reiches N, Roseman J M 1981 Clinical and biochemical studies on methylxanthine-related fibrocystic disease. Surgery 90: 299–304

Montgomery A C V, Palmer B V, Biswas S, Monteiro J C M P 1979 Treatment of severe cyclical mastalgia. Journal of the Royal Society of Medicine 72: 489–491

Nichols S, Waters W E, Wheeler M J 1980. Management of female breast disease by Southampton general practitioners. British Medical Journal 281: 1450–1453

Peters F, Hilgarth M, and Breckwoldt M 1982 The use of bromocriptine in the management of non-puerperal mastitis. Archives of Gynaecology 233: 23–29

Peters F, Pickardt C R, Zimmermann G, Breckwoldt M, 1981 PRL, TSH and thyroid hormones in benign breast disease. Klinische Wochenschrift 59: 403–407

Preece P E, Mansel R E, Hughes L E 1978 Mastalgia: Psychoneurosis or Organic Disease? British Medical Journal 1: 29–30

Preece P E, Mansel R E, Bolton P M, Hughes L E, Baum M, Gravelle I H 1976 Clinical syndromes of mastalgia. Lancet 2: 670–673

Preece P E, Baum M, Mansel R E, Webster, D J T, Fortt R W, Gravelle I H, Hughes L E 1982 Importance of mastalgia in operable breast cancer. British Medical Journal 284: 1299–1300

Preece P E, Richards A R, Owen G M, Hughes L E 1975 Mastalgia and total body water. British Medical Journal 4: 498–500

Read G F, Bradley J A, George W D, Wilson D W, Griffiths K 1985 Evaluation of luteal phase salivary progesterone levels in women with benign breast disease or primary breast cancer. European Journal of Cancer and Clinical Oncology 21: 9–17

Renwick S 1979 Modern management of benign mammary dysplasia Medical Journal of Australia 1: 562–566

Ricciardi I, Ianniruberto A 1979 Tamoxifen induced regression of benign breast lesions. Obstetrics and Gynaecology 54: 80–84

Sitruk-Ware L, Sterkers N, Mowszowicz I, Mauvais-Jarvis P 1977 Inadequate corpus luteal function in women with benign breast disease. Journal of Clinical Endocrinology and Metabolism 44: 771–774

Tietze A 1921 Ueber eine eigerhartige Haufung von Fallen mit Dystrophie der Rippenknorpel. Berliner Klinische Wochenschrift 30: 829–831

Urban J A 1963 Excision of the major duct system of the breast Cancer 16: 516–20

Wilson M C, Sellwood R A 1976 Therapeutic value of a supporting brassiere in mastodynia British Medical Journal 2:90

Wisbey J R, Kumar S, Mansel R E, Preece P E, Pye J K, Hughes L E 1983 Natural history of breast pain Lancet II 17: 672–4

5 Viral and cellular oncogenes a— molecular basis for breast and other cancers

ASHLEY R. DUNN

Cancer Research, like other areas of scientific endeavour, is prone to long phases of steady progress intermingled with shorter bursts of inspired achievement. By any standards, the last 5 years has witnessed a veritable torrent of information brought about as a direct and inevitable consequence of a technical revolution in molecular biology coupled with major advances in the techniques of gene transfer.

Introduction

While cancer is a disease which we recognise at the cellular level, it has a genetic basis. It probably starts with a limited number of primary changes in key cellular genes concerned with growth control and is followed by a cascade of secondary and subsequent genetic events. It seems likely that many of these latter events are simply by-products playing no direct role in the initiation of cancer; rather they contribute to the overall phenotype of the cancer cell.

Until recently a somewhat pessimistic view, shared by many, was that the identification of cancer genes (oncogenes) might be next to impossible. Recent research has cast these doubts aside; cancer genes have been recognised as components of both normal and cancer cells. We are now beginning to appreciate their role in normal cellular growth and development and in the profound consequences of genetic mutations which affect their structure and regulation (for recent reviews see Bishop, 1983a & 1983b; Weinberg, 1983)

This short essay is designed to capture the interest of clinicians who sense the excitement of recent discoveries but who have been unable to indulge themselves in the detail of individual reports and contributions. I can hope to give no more than a flavour of progress in the field often highlighting principles rather than detail.

Viruses and cancer

While viruses are not considered a major component of most human cancers they have long been implicated in several types of naturally arising cancers in animals. Consequently, since the earliest days of cancer research, viruses have attracted considerable attention as laboratory reagents capable of inducing tumours in animals and of transforming normal tissue culture cells into cancer cells. As we shall see, much of our recently gained knowledge of the molecular basis of human cancer can be traced back to the efforts of tumour virologists since the beginning of this century.

How then, might tumour viruses 'transform' cells? At the outset we could imagine three obvious possible mechanisms. Firstly, the virus itself may include a cancer gene in its chromosome; following infection and integration into the host cell chromosome(s) the viral cancer gene would be expressed in concert with other cellular genes. Expression of the viral oncogene would initiate and maintain the 'transformed' phenotype. Secondly, viruses which themselves lack cancer gene(s) could transform cells by disrupting the expression of normal cellular genes, possibly by integration into, or close to, an important cellular gene i.e. by acting as an insertional mutagen. Thirdly, viruses might transform cells by a 'hit and run' mechanism; the virus may disrupt cellular gene expression but need not necessarily remain physically associated with a specific cellular locus.

While there is little compelling evidence for 'hit and run' transformation by viruses it has become clear that viruses *including* and *lacking* cancer genes can 'transform' some tissue culture cells and initiate tumour development in the appropriate animal. Furthermore, the cancer genes carried by some transforming viruses and the cellular genes affected by transforming viruses themselves lacking oncogenes, are very closely related.

Retroviruses and oncogenes

Retroviruses have RNA as their genetic material and in their simplest form, the so-called Slow Transforming Retroviruses, comprise three genes (Fig. 5.1). Two of these genes encode structural information and the third an enzyme, RNA dependent DNA polymerase (reverse transcriptase), for converting their RNA genome into proviral DNA. Some retroviruses have evolved despite suffering deletions in their replication genes and consequently are themselves only able to replicate in the presence of complementing helper virus. Certain replication defective retroviruses, have been shown to include a supplementary gene (viral oncogene or v-onc) which in many cases confers on these viruses the ability to transform cultured cells with high efficiency and lead to tumour development upon injection into laboratory animals—hence their general name, the acute transforming retroviruses (Fig. 5.1). The origin of these supplementary genes for many years remained obscure until the discovery that normal Avian and Mammalian cellular DNA includes a gene very closely related to the oncogene of Rous sarcoma virus (Stehelin et al,

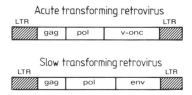

Fig. 5.1 *Retroviral genome structure.* The slow transforming retroviruses include 3 genes (gag, pol and env) bounded on each side by a long terminal repeat (LTR) which includes all of the regulatory sequences for expression of viral genes. The actue transforming retroviruses are often found to have incurred a deletion in one or more of their replication genes and concommitantly acquired a transduced cellular gene (see text).

1976). This discovery has now been extended to other acute transforming retroviruses: to date about 20 such cellular genes have been identified using retroviral genes as probes. In several cases, a detailed analysis of both viral and cellular genes has revealed close identity and led to the inescapable conclusion that specific cellular genes were 'captured' (transduced) during viral evolution. For these acutely transforming viruses, at least, transformation in some way arises by integration and expression of a viral gene closely related to a gene already present in the target cell.

How then do slow transforming retroviruses such as Avian Leukosis Virus (ALV) which lack a traditional oncogene convert 'normal' fibroblasts into cancer cells and lead to tumour development when injected into chickens. Studies of the DNA of several virally induced lymphomas of chickens has revealed the presence of an integrated proviral insertion close to the cellular homologue of the myc oncogene of MC29 virus (Fig. 5.2). In ALV induced lymphoma and presumably in tumours involving other slow transforming retroviruses, the virus acts as an insertional mutagen and neoplasia arises

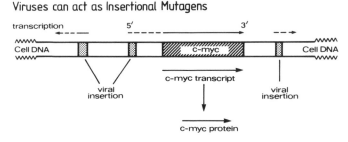

Fig. 5.2 *Viruses can act as insertional mutagens.* The slow transforming retroviruses transform cells, or induce tumours in animals, by integrating their proviral DNA into the cellular chromosome near to a cellular oncogene (in this example c-myc). In this diagrammatic representation the 3 stippled boxes (viral insertion) represent the alternative sites of integration of viral sequences and their transcriptional orientation is indicated by arrows. Transcription of c-myc is left to right. The proviral insertion immediately left of c-myc could influence c-myc expression by providing a novel transcriptional start site leading to the synthesis of a hybrid mRNA (and possibly a hybrid protein) comprising both viral and cellular information. In the case of either of the two outer viral insertions it is more likely that the level of c-myc transcription is altered either by the influence of a transcriptional enhancer contained within the LTR, or by dislocating the cellular regulatory elements which control normal c-myc transcription.

directly or indirectly as a result of altered expression of a cellular oncogene. Importantly, in the case of many individual tumours the nature of the viral insertion excludes the possibility of the synthesis of a novel hybrid mRNA and protein (see caption to Fig. 5.2). It now appears that a powerful element called a 'transcriptional-enhancer' is an important component of the regulatory sequences (located in the long terminal repeat) of several retroviruses which influences the natural promoter of the cellular myc gene leading to increased myc transcription. Apparently elevated expression of c-myc is a key event in the genesis of these tumours.

In summary, retroviruses can convert normal cells into cancer cells by donating a viral oncogene to the cell or by disturbing the expression of a normal cellular gene. In both cases the gene may be ancestrally related.

Human oncogenes and multistep carcinogenesis

In its simplest form a tumour represents an expanding clone of developmentally arrested cells. Unlike the cells from which they arise, cancer cells have lost their ability to respond to the normal stimuli (growth factors) which control the balance between cell divisions of self-renewal and those of differentiation. In this simple scheme, cancer represents a breakdown in the fundamental mechanisms that underlie normal growth. It follows then that in order to understand the genetic basis of cancer we must identify the genes whose products govern controlled growth, to understand the way in which they are regulated and to adapt these findings into the framework of cancer development established by cell biologists and epidemiologists.

In 1979 researchers at the Massachusetts Institute of Technology reasoned that if cancer were controlled by expression of 'cancer genes' then normal cells might be converted to cancer cells by transferring the DNA from one cell type to another. Purified DNA was isolated from fibroblasts that had been transformed into a tumour cell line by exposure to a chemical carcinogen. Using sensitive techniques of gene transfer, cultured NIH 3T3 fibroblasts were exposed to this tumour DNA; two weeks later foci of transformed cells appeared which were subsequently shown to give rise to tumours when transplanted into mice (Shih et al, 1979). Apparently then the transforming principle (oncogene) was encoded in the DNA of the original tumour cells and behaved as a dominant gene(s) in the recipient cell. The existence of transforming sequences was subsequently demonstrated in the DNA of a large number of different human tumours and tumour cell lines (Cooper, 1982). Several of these transforming principles have now been isolated by molecular cloning. In each case a simple fundamental truth has emerged. Each of them is closely related to a gene present in the chromosome of normal cells and furthermore, in several cases, this gene has been shown to be the cellular homologue of the viral oncogene of an acute transforming retrovirus.

Clearly, oncogenes present in tumours and presumably in part controlling the cancer phenotype (activated oncogenes) must differ from their normal

cellular counterparts in some fundamental way. Several mechanisms underlying oncogene activation have been established, some of them derived from
direct structural comparison of activated and normal cellular oncogenes and
others from laboratory experimentation. Firstly some, but not all, cellular
oncogenes can be converted into transforming factors by genetically linking
them to powerful viral regulatory sequences ensuring their over-expression
when established in hitherto normal cells. The levels of mRNA corresponding
to the cellular oncogene are accordingly higher and the cells behave like their
transformed counterparts. Several human tumours have apparently developed
as a result of high levels of expression of cellular oncogenes and in many cases
this has occurred as a result of gene amplification. The myc proto-oncogene
has been amplified 30–50 times in both a promyelocytic leukaemic cell line,
HL-60 (Collins & Groudine, 1982), and a neuroendocrinal colonic tumour
(Alitalo et al, 1983). Similarly proto-oncogene amplification has been
noted in a human colon carcinoma cell line (Ki-ras) (McCoy et al, 1983), an
adrenocortical tumour of mice (Ki-ras) (Schwab et al, 1983), several human
neuroblastomas (N-myc) (Brodeur et al, 1983) and a human myelogenous
leukaemic cell line (c-abl) (Collins & Groudine, 1983).

A second mechanism of activation involves a disturbance of the oncogene
locus by translocation. It has been well established for many years that certain
malignancies are characterised by specific cytogenetic abnormalities (Sandberg,
1980), e.g. the Philadelphia chromosome in acute myelogenous leukaemia. In
several cases it appears that a cellular oncogene is associated with the point of
chromosome breakage (Fig. 5.3). Chromosome translocation serves to trans-
pose the oncogene to a new environment resulting in a disruption of c-onc
expression. In many cases increased transcription of the cellular oncogene has
been noted and implied as a contributing factor in the genesis of tumours.

Human Burkitts lymphoma is typically characterised by a balanced recipro-
cal translocation involving chromosomes 8 and 14 (Fig. 5.3a). The resulting
aberrant chromosome places the cellular myc (c-myc) oncogene (normally on
chromosome 8) in juxtaposition with the immunoglobulin heavy chain gene of
chromosome 14. The cross-over point has been precisely mapped in many
human tumours and in most cases occurs within 2000 base pairs of DNA from
c-myc. While c-myc transcription is elevated in some individual tumours it is
not obviously the case in all of them. It has recently been shown that c-myc
expression is tightly coupled to the cell cycle raising the alternative possibility
that rearrangement of the c-myc locus dislocates the elements which control
normal regulation resulting in constitutive expression of c-myc protein.

Another translocation is that which accounts for the Philadelphia chromosome characteristic of chronic human myelogenous leukaemia (Fig. 5.3b). The
aberrant chromosome results from a translocation involving chromosomes 9
and 22. Chromosome 9 carries cellular abl (c-abl, the human cellular analogue
of the Abelson murine leukaemia viral oncogene), and chromosome 22, the
lambda light-chain immunoglobulin gene. While enhanced expression of c-abl
has been observed in some leukaemic cell lines the question of whether c-abl
translocation is an obligatory step in the development of myeloid leukaemias
is in doubt since translocations involving variant chromosomes, not involving

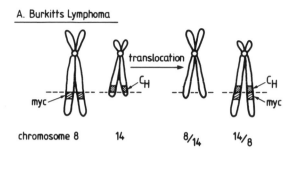

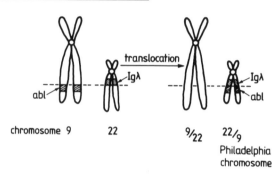

Fig. 5.3 *Chromosome translocations frequently associated with Burkitts Lymphoma and chronic myelogenous leukaemia.* Burkitts lymphoma (A) and chronic myelogenous leukaemia (B) are each characterised by distinct chromosome abnormalities resulting from balanced chromosome translocations. In each case established cellular oncogenes have been mapped to the sites of chromosome exchange. Translocation results in their relocation adjacent to immunoglobulin genes.

chromosome 9, have been observed. As in the case of Burkitts lymphoma the possibility that specific translocations occur as a consequence rather than a cause of cancer cannot be dismissed. Clearly, in both Burkitts lymphoma and chronic myelogenous leukaemia the correlations with specific chromosome translocations must be relevant in some way but conclusive proof that these, or related, translocations are the primary malignant event is presently lacking.

Finally, activation can involve genetic mutation within the coding sequences of an oncogene which ultimately gives rise to an alteration in the structure of the oncogene product. The best example for this mechanism has been established from analysis of the 'ras' family of cellular oncogenes (corresponding to the oncogenes of certain sarcoma inducing viruses of animals). It is firmly established in the case of a human bladder carcinoma cell line T24/EJ that a simple point-mutation is responsible for the activated state of the Harvey-ras cellular oncogene. A single nucleotide change in DNA (a G to T transversion) causes a glycine, normally present at the 12th residue of the p21 ras protein, to be replaced by a valine (Tabin et al, 1983). Similarly, in a human lung carcinoma a mutation in the cellular Harvey ras gene affects amino acid 61 of the p21 protein. Further studies of human tumours coupled with in vitro mutagenesis experiments suggests that the codons specifying residues 12 and 61 represent critical sites which, when mutated, often generate oncogenic alleles. Point mutations at other locations within the cellular ras gene only serve to inactivate these genes instead of converting them into transforming onco-genes. In tumours involving mutant oncogenes the levels of expression are unaltered and presumably in these cases cancer development in some way involves the synthesis of an altered p21.

It is widely thought that cancer is a disease which develops as a result of several steps which accumulate over a period of many years—a scheme which invokes multiple compounding molecular events and which at face value is inconsistent with the sole effects of a single activated oncogene. Some light has recently been thrown on this apparent paradox. Cultured mouse NIH 3T3 fibroblast cells, commonly used for gene transfer experiments, are readily transformed by 'ras' oncogenes whereas primary or secondary cultures of rat embryo fibroblasts are not. The difference, it would seem, lies in the fact that NIH 3T3 cells which have been in culture for many years are immortalised, that is, they have an infinite capacity for self-renewal unlike primary cultures of rodent fibroblasts. Presumably certain cellular functions are operating in NIH 3T3 cells but not in the primary fibroblast cultures and thus the NIH 3T3 cells are sensitive to transformation by activated oncogenes. It was subsequently shown that the primary fibroblast cultures could in fact be trans-formed when two co-operating but distinct oncogenes were included in the transfection mixture: apparently one class of oncogenes is functionally equiv-alent to the supposed cellular functions active in the immortal NIH 3T3 cells and expression of the second oncogene leads to 'full' transformation. These experiments are, for the most part, satisfyingly consistent with the model of multi-stage carcinogenesis and give hope that we might soon understand all of the genes whose products contribute to the initiation and development of cancer.

Oncogenes and growth factors

We have seen that disturbances in cellular oncogene expression can lead to uncontrolled growth; it follows logically that the role of cellular oncogenes in normal cells concerns some aspect of normal growth. We can be quite confident that the role played by cellular oncogene products is an important one; the DNA sequence of cellular oncogenes has been conserved across a wide range of vertebrate and invertebrate species—a reliable and well established hallmark of importance.

Normal cellular growth and differentiation is controlled, in part, by a variety of specific polypeptide growth factors, e.g. epidermal growth factor (EGF) and nerve growth factor (NGF). These factors interact with specific cell surface receptors and somehow promote cellular DNA synthesis in specific tissues. In some cases growth factors are required not only for growth of certain progenitor cells but also for their survival. Interestingly certain retroviruses can rescue these cells from their total dependence on a growth factor raising the possibility that the transforming viruses encode proteins functionally analogous to the cellular growth factors.

In the last year this prediction has been at least partially fulfilled by the demonstration that the viral oncogene of Simian sarcoma virus (SSV) is very closely related to the cellular gene encoding platelet-derived growth factor (PDGF). Apparently the ancestral progenitor of SSV transduced the cellular PDGF locus and concomitantly acquired oncogenic capability. There is now direct evidence that the viral oncogene of SSV functions as a PDGF agonist and affects cell division by interacting with the PDGF receptor. Logically then we might predict that cells which express PDGF inappropriately may appear to lose growth control. Indeed, NIH 3T3 fibroblast cells exposed to PDGF acquire some of the morphological characteristics of transformed cells. Furthermore, some human tumour cell lines have recently been shown to express a PDGF-like molecule and this may well be a contributing factor to their tumourigeneic phenotype (Bowen-Pope et al, 1984).

It has long been established that tumour cells have a reduced requirement for exogenous growth factors. Compared to their normal counterparts tumour cells are able to grow in growth medium supplemented with reduced levels of serum (a rich natural source of growth factors). It seems that the tumour cells themselves express growth factors to which the same cells respond (Sporn & Todaro, 1980). Indeed, culture medium conditioned by the growth of virally transformed cells is able to support the growth of hitherto normal cells which transiently acquire the morphological characteristics of tumour cells. When the conditioned medium is replaced by standard growth medium the cells quickly assume the phenotypic appearance of normal cells. The tumour cell conditioned medium has been shown to contain molecules called tumour growth factors (TGFs) which confer the transformed phenotype on normal cells. Importantly these factors are not encoded by the transforming viruses but rather represent cellular genes activated as a consequence of the expression of viral genes. The TGFs are known to interact with the normal cellular receptor for epidermal growth factor and this in some way leads to the cells 'transformed' phenotype.

A further link between oncogenes and the cellular pathways involving growth factors has recently been established by the demonstration that some oncogenes are structurally related to the growth factor receptors themselves. The cellular oncogene acquired by the progenitor of the avian erythroblastosis virus (AEV), the erb B oncogene, has strong amino acid sequence homology with a part of the EGF receptor. The significance of this observation is presently unclear since the precise role played by receptors in growth factor mediated cell division is somewhat equivocal. One possibility is that the growth factor serves to activate the receptor which in turn initiates intracellular messages involved in stimulating cell division. Certain similarities have been noted between the substrate specificites of growth factor receptor and oncogene products which may indicate a common metabolic pathway in growth and transformation.

In summary there is mounting evidence to suggest that one of the stages in tumourigenesis involves the inappropriate expression (including qualitative alterations) of certain genes whose products control the various steps in cellular growth, i.e. the growth factor itself, the specific cell surface receptor or the intracellular events which lead to the initiation of DNA synthesis. The factors may be encoded by oncogenes or induced indirectly as a consequence of oncogene expression.

Concluding remarks

I have discussed the crucial role played by cellular oncogenes in the disruption of normal growth and have also pointed to the vital role of oncogene products in the processes of normal growth and differentiation. At first sight it is difficult to see how our new found knowledge could be used to devise schemes whereby cellular oncogenes, or their products, might be inactivated in tumour cells but not simultaneously in normal cells. Over the coming years this problem will form the basis of very many research programmes.

REFERENCES

Alitalo K, Schwab M, Lin C C, Varmus H E, Bishop J M 1983 Homogeneously staining chromosomal regions contain amplified copies of an abundantly expressed cellular oncogene (c-myc) in malignant neuroendocrine cells from a human colon carcinoma. Proceedings of the National Academy of Science 80: 1707–1711
Bishop J M 1983a Cellular oncogenes and retroviruses. Annual Review of Biochemistry 52: 301–354
Bishop J M 1983b Cancer genes come of age. Cell 32: 1018–1020
Bowen-Pope D F, Vogel A, Ross P 1984 Production of platelet-derived growth factor-like molecules and reduced expression of platelet-derived growth factor receptors accompany transformation by a wide spectrum of agents. Proceedings of the National Academy of Science 81: 2396–2400
Brodeur G M, Seeger R C, Schwab M, Varmus H E and Bishop J M 1984 Amplification of N-myc in untreated human neuroblastomas correlates with advanced disease stage. Science 224: 1121–1124
Collins S, Groudine M 1982 Amplification of endogenous myc-releated DNA sequences in a human myeloid leukemia cell line. Nature (London) 298: 679–681
Collins S, Groudine M T 1983 Rearrangement and amplification of c-abl sequences in the human chronic myelogenous leukemia cell line K-562. Proceedings of the National Academy of Science 80: 4813–4817
Cooper G M 1982 Cellular transforming genes. Science 217: 801–806
Downward J, Yarden Y, Mayes E, Scrace G, Totty N, Stockwell P et al 1984 Close similarity of epidermal growth factor receptor and v-erb-B oncogene protein sequences. Nature (London) 307: 521–527
Land H, Parada L F, Weinberg R A 1983 Cellular oncogenes and multistep carcinogenesis. Science 222: 771–778
McCoy M S, Toole J J, Cunningham J M, Chang E H, Lowy D R, Weinberg R A 1983 Characterization of a human colon/lung carcinoma oncogene. Nature 302: 79–81
Sandberg A A (ed) 1980 The Chromosomes in Human Cancer and Leukemia. Elsevier/North-Holland, Amsterdam
Schwab M, Alitalo K, Varmus H E, Bishop J M, George D 1983 A cellular oncogene (c-Ki-ras) is amplified, overexpressed, and located within karyotypic abnormalities in mouse adrenocortical tumour cells. Nature (London) 303: 497–501
Shih C, Shilo B, Goldfarb M, Dannenberg A, Weinberg R A 1979 Passage of phenotypes of chemically transformed cells via transfection of DNA and chromatin. Proceedings of the National Academy of Science 76: 5714–5718

Sporn M B and Todaro G J 1980 Autocrine secretion and malignant transformation of cells. New England Journal of Medicine 303: 878–880

Stehelin D, Varmus H E, Bishop J M and Vogt P K 1976 DNA related to the transforming gene(s) of avian sarcoma viruses is present in normal avian DNA. Nature 260: 170–173

Tabin C J, Bradley S M, Bargmann C I, Weinberg R A, Papageorge A G, Scolnick E M, Dhar R, Lowy D R, Change E H 1983 Mechanism of activation of a human oncogene. Nature (London) 300: 143–149

Weinberg R A 1983 A molecular basis of cancer. Scientific American November: 102–116

Yunis J J 1983 The chromosomal basis of human neoplasia. Science 221: 227–236

6 The identification of patients at increased risk of breast cancer

N. F. BOYD

Introduction

The clinician who wishes to determine the risk of developing breast cancer faced by a particular patient is likely to find the literature dealing with the subject frustrating. While clinicians are concerned with individual patients, the epidemiologic literature is concerned almost entirely with groups of subjects. Clinicians and patients wish to obtain estimates of actual risk, while the literature cites mainly relative risks, and while patients may possess several attributes, each associated with an increase or decrease in risk, the literature seldom deals with the simultaneous effects of more than one variable on the risk of breast cancer. Furthermore, although the incidence of breast cancer increases strikingly with increasing age, and age must therefore be taken into account in assessing risk for an individual, the effects of risk factors at different ages are in general not known.

Nevertheless, an understanding of the literature, and of the methods used by epidemiologists to assess risk factors, may be useful for several reasons. It will allow the clinician to identify those data that are suitable for the estimation of risk for individuals, and to avoid the inappropriate use of information that is not suitable for this purpose. Such an understanding will also allow the clinician to follow progress in the field, and to assess the credibility of claims concerning new risk factors.

The purpose of this paper will not be to describe exhaustively the factors that influence risk of breast cancer, which have been the subject of several reviews (MacMahon et al, 1973; Kelsey, 1979; Kalache & Vessey, 1982), but rather to appraise critically the evidence that known risk factors can identify a group at increased risk of breast cancer. Particular emphasis will be placed on those factors that may be reversible. Although it seems likely that intervention directed at changing risk will be a subject for research for some time, it is of special importance because the recognition of individuals at increased risk is of little value unless their risk can be reduced in some way.

Definition of risk

Decisions about causes of disease rest ultimately upon comparisons of risk. The risk of developing disease in those exposed to a putative cause or risk factor is compared with the risk of disease in those not so exposed. The compared risks are often divided one by the other, to yield a single numerical expression, the *relative risk* (MacMahon & Pugh, 1970). Table 6.1 illustrates the method of calculating relative risk for the two research designs most commonly used for examining aetiologic associations. In *cohort* studies, individuals free of the disease under consideration, for present purposes breast cancer, are classified according to the presence or absence of the risk factor of interest, for example a family history of the disease, and then followed forward in time and observed for the development of breast cancer. The risk of developing breast cancer in those with a family history is then given by the number with a family history who develop breast cancer divided by the total number who had a family history of the disease (a/a + b in Table 6.1). Individuals without a family history are similarly followed and the risk of breast cancer in this group expressed in a similar calculation (c/c + d in Table 6.1). In some cohort studies the risk of disease in non-exposed subjects is not observed directly but is estimated from the risks of disease in a similarly aged group of individuals in the general population using population based statistics.

The relative risk of breast cancer associated with a family history of the disease is then calculated by the ratio of the two rates (a/a + b ÷ c/c + d). Relative risks in excess of unity thus imply that the risk factor is associated with an increase in risk, and if less than unity a decrease in risk.

Because cohort studies require that large numbers of individuals are followed for extended periods of time, aetiologic associations are often investigated with a case control method which requires no period of observation, and a smaller number of subjects than a cohort study for a given statistical power (Schlesselman, 1982).

In contrast to cohort studies, case control start by identifying subjects with breast cancer (the cases) and a comparison group without the disease (the controls). The frequency of antecedant exposure to the risk factor of interest is then compared in the two groups. Because of the way in which subjects are selected, risk of disease in exposed and non exposed subjects cannot be calculated directly, but can be estimated from the ratio of the odds of exposure in the cases and controls, an expression that is often referred to as relative risk but is more correctly called an odds ratio or rate ratio. This expression is calculated from Table 6.1 by (a/c ÷ b/d or ad/cb).

Table 6.1 Breast cancer: definition of risk

	Exposed Yes	No
Present	a	c
Absent	b	d
	a + b	c + d

Case control studies are generally thought to be more susceptible to bias than cohort studies, and, when available, evidence from cohort studies is thus generally given greater weight (Spitzer & Ibrahim, 1979). Criteria for assessing whether the associations revealed by aetiologic studies are likely to be causal have been suggested by Hill (1965).

Risk factors for breast cancer

Demographic, reproductive, and anthropometric risk factors

Table 6.2 lists the demographic, reproductive, and anthropometric variables that have been associated consistently with differences in breast cancer risk. The largest differences in risk are associated with age and country of residence (Doll et al, 1976). The risk in North America of a women developing breast cancer before age 70 is approximately 1 in 14. However, the annual risk at ages 35–39 is approximately 53 per 100 000, 156 per 100 000 at ages 45–49, and 228 per 100 000 at ages 65–69 (Third National Cancer Survey, 1975). The large differences in breast cancer risk associated with country of residence, although of great interest to students of aetiology, and an important source of information concerning possible strategies for intervention (see below), is of little concern to the clinician whose practice will be influenced by the prevalence of disease in the environment where he works.

The remaining variables shown in Table 6.2 are much less strongly associated with breast cancer risk, with relative risks of the order of two or less (MacMahon et al, 1973; Kelsey, 1979; Kalache & Vessey, 1982). Early age at first birth has been consistently associated with a decrease in breast cancer risk. It appears that a full-term pregnancy is necessary for this protective effect, and that pregnancies terminating in abortion may be associated with increased risk. Breast cancer risk has also long been recognized to decline with increasing parity. However, this effect appears to be explained at least in part by the tendency for high parity to be associated with early age at first birth. The effect of parity on breast cancer risk is thus likely explained by the effect of age at first birth. Similarly, breast feeding and parity are associated, and breast feeding does not appear to reduce the risk of breast cancer after parity has been

Table 6.2 Demographic, reproductive and anthropometric risk factors for breast cancer

Risk factor	Higher risk	Lower risk	Relative risk
Age	Older	Younger	5–7
Country of Residence	N. America	Asia	
	— Europe	— Africa	5–7
Age at First Birth	Older	Younger	2–3
Number of Births	None	Some	2–3
Age at Menarche	Earlier	Later	1.5–2
Age at Menopause	Later	Earlier	1.5–2
Oophorectomy	None	When Young	1.5–2
Body Weight	Increased	Decreased	1.5–3
Height	Increased	Decreased	1.5–3

taken into account. Early menarche and late menopause are both associated with an increased risk of breast cancer. Oophorectomy appears to reduce breast cancer risk, the protective effect being greater the earlier in life that it is carried out.

An increase in body weight has been shown by several studies to be associated with a moderate increase in the relative risk of breast cancer (DeWaard & Halewijn, 1974; DeWaard, Baandersvan-Halewign, Huizinga, 1964; Wynder et al, 1960; Valaoras et al, 1969), most consistently in postmenopausal women. Height, and weight for height ratios such as the Quetelet Index, have also been associated with an increased risk in some studies.

Family history

Several studies have shown that the risk of developing breast cancer for women with first degree relatives with the disease is two to three times that of women with unaffected relatives. Anderson (1973) has shown that the degree of risk is strongly influenced by the menopausal status of the affected relative at the time the disease developed, by whether the disease was unilateral or bilateral, and by whether the affected relative was a mother or a sister. The risk of breast cancer was found to be increased only in those whose relatives had developed breast cancer while premenopausal, and no increase in risk was found for those whose relatives developed the disease when postmenopausal. The risk increased five-fold for those whose relatives had bilateral disease, and nine-fold for those whose relatives had developed bilateral disease while premenopausal. The relatives of patients who developed unilateral breast cancer when post-menopausal showed an excess risk of only 1.2. Anderson has further shown that the risk of breast cancer for the sisters of patients who develop the disease before the menopause is substantially increased if the mother also had premeno-pausal breast cancer.

Quantitative estimates of risk for first degree relatives at various ages have recently been provided by the work of Ottman and her colleagues (1983). This work is based upon observation of a cohort of mothers and sisters of patients with breast cancer in Los Angeles, and the results should therefore be applied cautiously in other parts of the world. Patients were classified according to their age at diagnosis, and whether the disease was unilateral of bilateral. Table 6.3 summarizes a portion of their results and shows the risk according to age, for sisters of patients with breast cancer, who were classified according to age at diagnosis. Thus at age 30 the sister of a patient whose breast cancer was diagnosed before the age of 40, and who has bilateral breast cancer, has a 23% chance of developing breast cancer before the age of 50 and is virtually certain to develop the disease before age 70.

Despite some uncertainties concerning estimates of risk based upon relatively small numbers of cases, these data comprise the only information presently available that provides a quantitative basis for counselling patients about risk of breast cancer.

Although in some circumstances associated with substantial risk, a family history of breast cancer affects relatively few people. In the Health Insurance Plan of New York study 9 of 203 patients with breast cancer gave a history

Table 6.3 Risk of breast cancer diagnosis at given age ranges for sisters of breast cancer patients by age at diagnosis and number of sides affected in patients

Sisters' age interval		Diagnosis in patients						
		Bilateral premenopausal			Unilateral premenopausal			Unilateral post-menopausal
Beginning	End	($\leqslant 40$)*	(41–50)	Total	($\leqslant 40$)	(41–50)	Total	($\geqslant 51$)
30	40	0.077	0.049	0.057	0.037	—	0.007	—
	50	0.235	0.090	0.121	0.079	0.041	0.048	0.052
	60	0.592	0.305	0.388	0.079	0.070	0.074	0.093
	70	0.999	0.305	0.511	0.079	0.070	0.074	0.184

* Age at diagnosis of patients.
From Ottman et al (1983)

of the disease in a mother, and 17 of 203 a history of breast cancer in a sister (Shapiro et al, 1973).

Effects of combining risk factors

The risk factors reviewed thus far have the shortcoming of either, as with the reproductive and anthropometric variables, having a relatively weak influence upon risk, or as in the case with family history, being so uncommon that only a small proportion of breast cancer risk can be explained by them. Nevertheless, it seems possible that individuals with several attributes, each associated with an increase in risk, may be at greater risk than those with only one such factor, and that the identification of such individuals may define a high risk group.

This question has been examined in two large cohort studies in which risk factors were documented at entry to the study, and the individuals then followed and observed for the development of breast cancer. In one, the Health Insurance Plan of New York's randomized controlled trial of screening for breast cancer with mammography, data on risk factors were obtained from 20 000 women who responded to the invitation to be screened (Shapiro, 1973). In the other, information about risk factors was obtained from 5000 women volunteers who were enrolled in a prospective study of breast cancer risk factors on the island of Guernsey (Farewell, 1977).

In the Health Insurance Plan study, after an extensive examination of the risks of breast cancer associated with single variables, women who had ever married (who comprised 93% of the total population) were classified according to whether they had three or more, or less than three of the following variables: menarche at age less than 15; less than three pregnancies; first pregnancy at age 30 or over; prior breast conditions; one or more sisters with breast cancer. During the 5 years that this large population of subjects was followed, 203 breast cancers developed. Thirty-three per cent of these cancers were in women with three or more of the risk factors enumerated, and 67% of the cancers were in those with less than three risk factors. It was concluded that the five risk factors examined did not identify a population that could be made the principal target of a screening programme.

Farewell examined four risk factors, age at menarche, family history, age at first birth, and etiocholanolone excretion. Each of these variables made a significant improvement in the prediction made by the remaining three variables of who would develop breast cancer, and no other variable was found which provided any further improvements. The presence of two or more risk factors correctly identified 37 (82%) of the 45 women who developed breast cancer in this cohort, but included 55% of the larger population of 770 women who did not develop breast cancer. Three (7%) of the women who developed breast cancer had four or more risk factors, compared to 28 (2%) of the women who did not develop breast cancer. It was concluded that these risk factors did not allow the identification of a group who could be the subjects of selective screening.

Mammographic patterns

Wolfe has described differences in breast cancer risk associated with different appearances of the breast parenchyma on mammography (Wolfe, 1967; Wolfe, 1967a; Wolfe, 1977, Wolfe, 1976; Wolfe et al, 1982) a breast parenchyma comprised of fat (designated N1 in Wolfe's classification) is reported to be associated with the lowest risk of breask cancer, whereas the highest risk of breast cancer is associated with radiologic evidence of dysplasia (designated DY by Wolfe). Wolfe has also described intermediate levels of risk in association with the presence of prominent ducts in the breast parenchyma on mammography. The large differences in breast cancer risk reported to be associated with these various radiologic appearances have prompted several other investigators to examine mammographic patterns as indicators of risk for breast cancer with results that are summarized in Table 6.4. The table includes all of the reports that used Wolfe's terminology for classification and were published in the English language between 1976 and 1983. The reports are classified according to their research architecture, as prevalence surveys, cohort or case control studies. (Prevalence surveys are those that classified patients undergoing mammography according to pattern and whether or not cancer was detected). Several studies incorporated both prevalence and cohort components in their design. Wolfe's own studies are omitted.

The table shows a very wide distribution of estimates of relative risk ranging from 0.06 to infinity, both statistically significant but diametrically opposed associations. Overall, 12 studies found an increased breast cancer risk associated with the DY pattern, 4 a decreased risk, and 7 failed to find a statistically significant association between pattern and breast cancer risk. We have assessed these conflicting results by examining their adherence to commonly accepted methodologic standards for the investigation of causal relationships. The nine standards for which the studies were examined were: a description of the way in which the study population have been assembled, the avoidance of referral bias in assembling the subjects, 'blind' reading of films, assessment of observer variation in classification, adjusting for age and other risk factors for breast cancer in the analysis of risk, and in the case of cohort studies, specifying the duration of follow-up, the frequency of examination, and specifying how losses to follow-up were managed. We found a strong association between the standards adopted by a study and the results obtained (Boyd et al, 1984).

Table 6.4 Relative risk of breast cancer with DY pattern according to study design

Author (ref)	Prevalence survey	Cohort	Author (ref)	Case Control
Egan 1977	0.24[1,4]	8.16[1,2,3]	Mendell 1977	1.27[1,5]
Krook 1978	1.52[1]	7.34[1,3]	Peyster 1977	0.61[1,4]
Egan 1979	0.46[2,4]	2.93[1,2,3,6]	Rideout 1977	0.06[1,4]
Threatt 1980	∞[1,3,7]	∞[1,3,7]	Wilkinson 1977	5.8[3]
Tabar 1982	1.60[1]	1.23[1,2]	Hainline 1978	7.2[3]
Brebner 1978	1.19	—	Ernster 1980	0.72[1]
Janzon 1982	1.50[3,5]	—	Brisson 1982	1.9[3]
Krook 1978	—	7.75[3]	Gravelle 1980	4.93[1,3]
Moskowitz 1980	—	1.20[1]	Boyd 1982	3.30[3]

[1] Relative risk calculated by present authors.
[2] Followup information incomplete or absent.
[3] Significant increase in breast cancer risk with DY pattern ($p < 0.05$).
[4] Significant decrease in breast cancer risk with DY pattern ($p < 0.05$).
[5] Relative risk of DY + P2 versus P1 + N1.
[6] Calculation based upon number of examinations, not number of patients.
[7] ∞ relative risk arises because no cases of breast cancer were observed in patients with the N1 pattern.
   From Boyd et al (1984).

Among nine cohort and case control studies that found a statistically significant association between mammographic pattern and breast cancer risk, all met at least four standards, whereas only two of the six 'negative' cohort or case control studies met as many as four standards. Among prevalence surveys the association between methods and results was less striking, but several 'negative' prevalence surveys were associated with 'positive' cohort studies employing the same group of patients. These results indicate that methodologic differences between studies contribute substantially to the controversy surrounding this subject. Studies that followed the usual scientific methods employed in the epidemiologic investigation of risk have generally confirmed an association between mammographic pattern and breast cancer risk. Cohort studies, usually considered to be the strongest design for the evaluation of risk have most consistently confirmed this relationship, but is should be noted that the five positive cohort studies referred to in the table comprise only three distinct populations of patients.

Some authors, while confirming the association of the DY pattern with breast cancer risk, have concluded that the observation is of little practical importance because the quantitative association observed is not strong enough to permit selective screening with mammography (Tabar and Dean, 1982; Janzon et al, 1982). While caution concerning selective screening on the basis of mammographic patterns seems entirely appropriate the importance of the observed association may lie more in the influence it may have in guiding future research into the aetiology of breast cancer.

Histology and cytology as indicators of breast cancer risk

The relationship of benign breast disease to breast cancer risk has long been debated by surgeons, pathologists, and epidemiologists. Progress in the subjects has been hampered by lack of a generally agreed definition for benign disease of the breast (Love et al, 1982). Some authors have defined the entity by a history of a previous breast biopsy, thus identifying a very heterogenous group of patients; some have used the designation 'fibrocystic disease', a term that encompasses a wide variety of epithelial and stromal changes that do not necessarily connote disease; while others have adopted a more rigorous approach that describes the type of histologic change in the breast epithelium of the individuals being studied. The subject of precancerous lesions in the human breast has recently been reviewed by Lagious (1983).

Wellings and Jensen (1973) have described a method of classifying the morphology of the breast epithelium of the terminal ductal lobular unit. This anatomical site has been shown by these workers, using a three-dimensional study of whole breast sections from subjects with breast cancer, to be the location where the smallest independent foci of ductal carcinoma in situ were observed. Their classification describes a continuum of morphologic change from normal epithelium, through hyperplasia without atypia, hyperplasia with atypia of increasingly severe grade, to carcinoma in situ and invasive cancer. Table 6.5 shows the frequency of some of these changes in the breasts of subjects with breast cancer, and a comparison group of subjects without breast cancer who were examined at autopsy. Hyperplasia of the terminal duct epithelium was 22 times more common in subjects with cancer, atypia four times more common, and ductal carcinoma in situ 68 times more common in the subjects with cancer. Black and Chabon (1969) have developed a similar method of grading mammary epithelium which also discriminates sharply between subjects with cancer and controls, and can be applied to ducts in any location in the breast.

Table 6.5 Lesions found in association with breast cancer

Epithelium	Average number per breast	
	Autopsy (n=183)	Breast cancer (n=107)
Normal	7.74	11.64
Hyperplasia	2.04	11.44
Mild Atypia	0.46	7.13
Moderate Atypia	0.18	3.31
C.I.S.*	0.08	5.45

* Carcinoma in situ
From Wellings et al (1975)

These approaches to the classification of breast epithelium have been shown to be associated with differences in breast cancer risk in two cohort studies based upon an initial classification of breast epithelium obtained on surgical biopsy and subsequent follow-up. However, it is not at present clear what sampling error might be involved in surgical biopsy. Thus if a biopsy shows atypical epithelium one can be sure that the patient has at least that level of change in the epithelium, but if the epithelium on biopsy is normal one cannot be sure whether another biopsy would reveal hyperplasia or atypia. Further, the reliability of the histologic classification between pathologists is not at present known.

Petrakis and co-workers (1982) have shown that breast fluid obtained from the nipple can provide information about breast cancer risk. Fluid is obtained using the method of Sartorious (1977) in which a plastic cup is placed over the nipple and suction applied by a 10 cc syringe connected to the cup by a short length of plastic tubing. In between 30 and 70% of subjects some fluid can be obtained in this way which contain cells, some of which resemble duct cells morphologically. Fluid is more often obtained from subjects with the demographic and reproductive risk factors referred to earlier, and the cells contained in the fluid are more often atypical in those with such risk factors. Cellular atypia in the nipple aspirate has also recently been shown (King et al, 1984) to be associated with cancer of the breast. Seventy per cent of subjects with breast cancer showed atypical cells in the aspirate compared to 54% of subjects without breast cancer but with atypical epithelium on biopsy and 24% of those without atypia on biopsy.

The role of screening

The evidence cited above shows that conventional demographic, reproductive and anthropometric variables do not define groups of individuals that can be made the sole target of a selective screening programme. In patients with a family history of breast cancer, specific risks can be calculated for the individual concerned. For patients at markedly increased risk there is little available data on the respective merits of careful follow-up and examination to detect cancers while still curable, versus prophylactic mastectomy. However, the decision as to what level of risk can be tolerated, and the severity of the loss incurred by mastectomy, is a highly personal one that is likely to vary greatly from one patient to another. The clinician faced with a patient at increased risk by virtue of a strong family history can perhaps best serve the patient's interests by ensuring that she understands the nature and magnitude of the risk involved, and is fully appraised of the available choices for management.

The data presently available on the risk associated with mammographic patterns, epithelial changes on biopsy, or nipple cytology, is still too incomplete to form the basis for a screening policy. These variables may nonetheless be useful as possible targets for intervention studies directed at the reduction of breast cancer risk.

Opportunities for intervention

The evidence that breast cancer, and other common malignancies, may be preventable has recently been reviewed by Doll and Peto (1981) and is derived in part from epidemiologic observations that show a striking international variation in breast cancer incidence and mortality. Breast cancer incidence and mortality are generally low in far Eastern and African countries, and high in North America and Europe (Doll et al, 1976).

Studies of migrants provide evidence that these international differences in breast cancer incidence are not due to genetic factors, but rather are attributable to environmental influences. Migrants moving from countries of low breast cancer incidence to high incidence countries eventually acquire the breast cancer incidence of the country to which they move (Buell, 1973; Haenzel & Kurihara, 1968).

There is considerable circumstantial evidence indicating that diet is an environmental factor closely associated with breast cancer risk which has been the subject of recent reviews (Reddy et al 1980; Carroll et al, 1968; Miller, 1976). Several workers have shown that the international variation of breast cancer incidence is strongly correlated with estimates of per capita fat consumption (Reddy et al, 1980; Carroll et al, 1968; Armstrong and Doll, 1975; Lea, 1966; Draser, 1973).

Analysis of changes in breast cancer incidence within countries also shows a positive correlation with changes in dietary fat consumption. For example, the rise in breast cancer incidence observed in Japan since 1950 has occurred at the same time as the adoption of a more Western style of life, including increased consumption of meat, eggs, and milk products (Hirayama, 1979).

The epidemiologic observations on human populations derive considerable support from experimental studies in animals. Tannenbaum & Silverstone (1957) have shown that the formation of mammary tumours in mice is promoted by obesity and retarded by caloric restriction, and that isocaloric diets high and low in fat are associated respectively with a high and low incidence of mammary tumours (Tannenbaum 1942). In studies with chemically induced mammary tumours in mice, Carroll and Khor (1975) have shown that dietary fat increases tumour formation only when given after tumour initiation, indicating that in this system, dietary fat acts as a tumour promoter.

Hypotheses concerning the relationship of diet to breast cancer risk, generated by either epidemiological observations or animal experimentation, need to be tested in humans before we can be assured of their relevance to human disease. Dietary intervention studies, in which a dietary change is made in a group of individuals who are then observed for a change in the frequency of cancer, are an attractively direct way of testing such hypotheses. Studies of this type, however, pose formidable methodologic difficulties. These include the relative infrequency of even the most common human tumours, and in consequence, the long periods of observation and large sample sizes required to detect an effect of dietary change upon cancer incidence.

An alternative strategy, that allows at least some of these problems to be circumvented, is to use a change in a lesion that is a precursor to cancer, rather than cancer itself, as the target measure for dietary intervention studies (Bruce et al, 1981).

To apply this strategy to breast cancer is of course necessary to identify a risk factor that is a suitable target for dietary intervention. None of the many well-documented risk factors for breast cancer, such as parity, age at first pregnancy, or family history of breast cancer, is susceptible to change in affected individuals, but other factors such as mammographic pattern, and histologic or cytologic changes, may be suitable targets for such intervention studies.

REFERENCES

Anderson D E 1973 Genetic study of breast cancer: identification of a high risk group. Cancer 34: 1090–1097

Armstrong B, Doll R 1975 Environmental factos and cancer incidence and mortality in different countries with special reference to dietary practices. International Journal of Cancer 15: 617–631

Black M M, Barclay T H C, Cutter S J, Hankey B F, Asire A J 1972 Association of atypical characteristics of benign breast lesions with frequent risk of breast cancer. Cancer 29: 338–343

Boyd N F, O'Sullivan B, Campbell J E, Fishell E, Simor I, Cooke G, Germanson T 1982 Bias and the association of mammographic parenchymal patterns with breast cancer. British Journal of Cancer 45: 179–184

Boyd, N F, O'Sullivan B, Fishell E, Simor I, Cooke G 1984 Mammographic patterns and breast cancer risk: methodologic standards and contradictory results. Journal of the National Cancer Institute 72: 1253–1259

Brebner D M, Epstein E E, Lange M 1978 Xerographic parenchymal patterns. Risk indicator for breast cancer? South African Medical Journal 54: 853–856

Brisson J, Sadowsky N L, Twaddle J A, Morrison A S, Cole P, Merletti F 1982 Mammographic features of the breast and breast cancer risk. American Journal of Epidemiology 115: 428–437

Bruce W R, Eyssen G M, Ciampi A, Dion D W, Boyd N F 1981 Strategies for dietary intervention studies in colon cancer. Cancer 47: 1121–1125

Buell P 1973 Changing incidence of breast cancer in Japanese—American women. Journal of the National Cancer Institute 51: 1479–1483

Carroll K K, Gammell E B, Plunkett E R 1968 Dietary fat and mammary cancer. Canadian Medical Association Journal 98: 590–594

Carroll K K, Khor H T 1975 Dietary fat in relation to tumori-genesis. Progress and Biochemical and Pharmacology 10: 308–354

Chaudary M A, Gravelle I H, Bulstrode J C, Wang D Y, Millis R R Hayward J L 1983 Breast parenchymal patterns in women with bilateral primary breast cancer. British Journal of Radiology 56: 703–706

DeWaard F, Halewijn E A B 1974 A prospective study in general practice on breast cancer risk in postmenopausal women. International Journal of Cancer 14: 153–160

Doll R, Peto R 1981 The causes of cancer: quantitative estimates of avoidable risks of cancer in the United States today. Journal of the National Cancer Institute 66: 1193–1265

Doll R, Muir C, Waterhouse J (eds) 1976 Cancer incidence in five continents. IARC Scientific Publication

Drasar B S, Irving D 1973 Environmental factors and cancer of the colon and breast. British Journal of Cancer 27: 167–172

Egan L, Mosteller C 1977 Breast cancer mammographic patterns. Cancer 40: 2087–2090

Egan R L, McSweeney M B 1979 Mammographic parenchymal patterns and risk of breast cancer. Radiology 133: 65–70

Ernster V I, Sack S T, Peterson C A, Schweitzer R J 1980 Mammographic parenchymal patterns and risk factors for breast cancer. Radiology 134: 617–620

Farewell V T 1977 The combined effect of breast cancer risk factors. Cancer 40: 931–936

Gravelle I H, Bustrode J C, Wang D Y, Hayward J L 1980 The relation between radiographic features and determinants of risk of breast cancer. British Journal of Cancer 53: 107–113

Haenzel W, Kurinara M 1968 Studies of Japanese migrants I. Mortality from cancer and other diseases among Japanese in the United States. Journal of the National Cancer Institute 40: 43–68

Hainline S, Myers L, McLelland R, Newll J, Gruggerman S, Shingleton W 1978 Mammographic patterns and risk of breast cancer. American Journal of Roentgenology 130: 1157–1158

Hill A B 1965 The environment and disease: Association of causation. Proceedings of the Royal College Society of Medicine 58: 295–300

Janzon L, Andersson I, Petersson H 1982 Mammographic patterns as indicators of risk of breast cancer. Raiology 143: 417–419

Kalache A, Vessey M 1982 Risk factors for breast cancer. In: Baum M (ed) Clinics in Oncology, Vol 1, No 3

Kelsey J L 1979 A review of the epidemiology of human breast cancer. In: Sartwell P E (ed) Epidemiologic Reviews, 1. Johns Hopkins University press, Baltimore p 74–109

Krook P M 1975 Mammographic parenchymal patterns as risk indicators for incident cancer in a screening program: An extended analysis. American Journal of Radiology 131: 1031–1035

Krook P M, Carlile T, Bush W, Hall M H 1978 Mammographic parenchymal patterns as a risk indicator for prevalent and incident cancer. Cancer 41: 1093–1097

King E B, Chew K L, Petrakis N L, Ernster V L 1983 Nipple aspirate cytology for the study of breast cancer precursors. Journal of the National Cancer Institute, 71: 1115–1121

Lagios M D 1983 Human breast precancer: current status cancer surveys, Vol 2, 3: 382–402

Lea A J 1966 Dietary factors associated with death rates from certain neoplasms in man. Lancet 2: 332–333

Love S M, Gelman R S, Silen W 1982 Fibrocystic 'disease' of the breast—a non-disease? New England Journal of Medicine, 307: 1010–1014

MacMahon B, Cole P, Brown J 1973 Etiology of Human Breast Cancer: A review. Journal of the National Cancer Institute, 50: 21–42

MacMahon B, Pugh T E 1970 Epidemiology. Principles and Methods. Little Brown and Company, Boston

Mendell L, Rosenbloom M, Naimark A 1977 Are breast patterns a risk index for breast cancer? A reappraisal. American Journal of Roentgenology 128:547

Miller A B 1977 Role of nutrition in the etiology of breast cancer. Cancer 39: 2704–2708

Moskowitz M, Gartside P, McLaughlin C 1980 Mammographic patterns as markers for high-risk benign breast disease and incident cancer. Radiology 134: 293–295

Ottman R, King M C, Pike M C, Henderson B E 1983 Practical guide for estimating risk for familial breast cancer. Lancet 556–558

Petrakis N L, Ernster V L, Sacks S T, King E B, Schweitzer R J, Hunt T K, King M C 1981 Epidemiology of breast fluid secretion: association with breast cancer risk factors and cerumen type. Journal of the National Cancer Institute, 67: 277–284

Peyster R G, Kalisher L, Cole P Mammographic parenchymal patterns and the prevalence of breast cancer. Radiology 125: 387–391

Reddy B S, Cohen L A, McCoy G D, Hill P, Weisburger J H, Wynder E L 1980 Nutrition and its Relationship to Cancer. In: Klein G, (ed) Advances in Cancer Research. Vol 32 Academic Press, New York

Rideout D F, Poon P Y 1977 Patterns of breast parenchyma on mammography. Journal of the Canadian Association of Radiology 28: 257–258

Sartorius D W, Smith H S, Morris P, Benedict D, Friesen L 1977 Cytologic evaluation of breast fluid in the detection of breast disease. Journal of the National Cancer Institute 59: 1073–1080

Schlesselman J J 1982 Case Control Studies. Design, Conduct, Analysis. Oxford University Press, Oxford

Shapiro S, Goldberg J, Venet L, Strax P 1973 Risk factors in breast cancer—a prospective study

Tabar L, Dean P B 1982 Mammographic parenchymal patterns. Risk indicator for breast cancer? Journal of the American Medical Association 247: 185–189

Tannenbaum A 1942 The genesis and growth of tumours IV. Effects of a high fat diet. Cancer Research 2: 468–475

Tannenbaum A, Silverstone H 1957 In: Raven R W (ed) Cancer Vol 1 p 306–334

The Third National Cancer Survey 1975 National Cancer Institute Monograph 41. DHEW Publication No. NIH 75–787, Bethesda

Threatt B, Norbeck J M, Ullman N S, Kummer R, Rosell P 1980 Association between mammographic parenchymal pattern classification and incidence of breast cancer. Cancer 45: 2550–2556

Valaoras V G, MacMahon B, Trichopoulos D 1969 Lactation and reproductive histories of breast cancer patients in greater Athens. International Journal of Cancer 4: 350–363

Wellings S R, Jensen H M, Marcum R G 1975 An atlas of syndrome pathology of the human breast with special preference to possible precancerous lesions. Journal of the National Cancer Institute 55: 231–273

Wilkinson E, Clopton C, Gordonson J, Green R, Hill A, Pike M C 1977 Mammographic parenchymal pattern and the risk of breast cancer. Journal of the National Cancer Institute 59: 1397–1400

Wolfe J N 1976 Breast patterns as an index of risk for developing breast cancer. American Journal of Roentgenology 126: 1130–1139

Wolfe J N, Albert S, Belle S, Salane M 1982 Breast parenchymal patterns: analysis of 332 incident breast carcinomas. American Journal of Roentgenology 138: 113–118

Wolfe J N 1967 Risk for breast cancer development determined by mammographic parenchymal pattern. Cancer 37: 2486–2492

Wolfe J N 1976 Breast parenchymal patterns and their changes with age Radiology 121: 545–552

Wolfe J N 1977 Risk of developing breast cancer determined by mammography. In: Wolfe J N (ed) Breast Cancer. Alan R. Liss, New York

Wynder E L, Bross J J, Hirayama T 1960 A study of the epidemiology of breast cancer 13: 559–601

Ibrahim M A 1979 The case control study: consensus and controversy. Journal of Chronic Disease 32:

7 Breast cancer genetics: definition of risk, patterns of inheritance, and management of patients and family members

MARY CLAIRE KING

Many breast cancer patients have mothers, sisters, or other relatives who have also suffered this disease. Very frequently, these patients ask whether their cancer may have been inherited. These women, and even breast cancer patients without affected relatives, also often ask whether their daughters may have inherited their susceptibility. These questions are difficult. The purpose of this chapter is to present some of the evidence on familial clustering and genetic inheritance of breast cancer. As we will see, each patient's question requires an individualized response. For most patients, breast cancer is not inherited, and they will not pass any risk on to their daughters. For other patients, breast cancer susceptability may have been inherited, and their daughters may be at increased risk. To assist surgeons with their patients' queries, we will explore two issues: firstly, in what families does breast cancer cluster and secondly, how is susceptibility to breast cancer inherited?

Familial aggregation of breast cancer: definition of risk

Breast cancer patients and their physicians are often the first to suggest that the disease may be familial. In order to test such an hypothesis, epidemiologic and statistical methods may be used to decide whether familial aggregation of the disease is real or due to chance co-occurrence of a common condition. We could conclude that breast cancer does aggregate in families when epidemiologic evidence indicates either that the incidence or prevalence of breast cancer among relatives of patients is higher than the incidence or prevalence of breast cancer among relatives of otherwise comparable, cancer-free controls or that a higher proportion of cases than controls have a relative with breast cancer.

An important methodological dilemma in the study of familial aggregation of breast cancer is the problem of disease heterogeneity. Relevant questions include whether certain subsets of breast cancer can be distinguished using clinical, epidemiologic, or genetic criteria, and whether families or individuals within families with different risks can be identified. Familial aggregation studies, in turn, can lead to insights about heterogeneity of breast cancer.

Just as breast cancer appears to constitute a clinically and etiologically heterogeneous group of diseases, so have laboratory experiments and epidemiological studies established a variety of environmental agents (various chemicals, certain viruses, and ionizing radiation) carcinogenic to mammary tissue in experimental animals or humans. Much work over the past few decades has helped elucidate the mechanisms by which these agents cause cancer (reviewed in Yuspa & Harris, 1982). The process by which these agents act, either by altering DNA in target cells (a process called initiation) or by enhancing cell multiplication (a process called promotion), are increasingly well understood. Animal experiments and epidemiologic and genetic studies also have presented convincing evidence that genetic susceptibility plays a role in carcinogenesis. For example, inbred strains of laboratory mice differ in their propensity to spontaneous mammary tumor formation. Also, different strains and species of animals differ in their susceptibility to chemical carcinogens. Some of these differences are explained by differences in metabolism of carcinogens.

The molecular genetics of breast cancer has proven extremely difficult. Many other human cancers are associated with chromosome abnormalities (Yunis, 1983), and recent work in molecular biology has demonstrated that oncogenes are involved in these rearrangements (Bishop, 1983). Oncogenes are human DNA sequences homologous to viral genes that cause cancer in animals and are therefore good candidates for a role in human oncogenesis. Work is in progress to elucidate the normal function of these genes in order to understand how alterations in their chromosomal positions cause cells to become cancerous. Furthermore, some families exhibit extraordinary risks of breast cancer, or of cancers of the breast and other sites, such as families with breast cancer, brain cancer, sarcoma, adrenocorticoid carcinoma, and leukemia (Shimke, 1978; Anderson, 1982). The existence and identification of such families has important implications for understanding the etiology of cancer and for rational counseling of cancer risk. Genetic susceptibility may be responsible for cancer aggregation in some of these high risk families. Moreover, progress has been made on specifying the mode of genetic inheritance in some of these families.

However, inasmuch as these high risk families are ascertained precisely because they contain many cases of breast cancer, they cannot be used to decide if familial aggregation is a regular feature of breast cancer. Numerous case-control and population-based studies have shown that breast cancer may aggregate in families (Anderson, 1982; King, 1982; Petrakis et al, 1982). Recent studies in the United States (Bain et al, 1980; Brinton et al, 1982, 1983; Ottman et al, 1983), Sweden (Adami et al, 1980, 1981) and Iceland (Tulinius et al, 1982) confirm that the risk of breast cancer to women with an affected mother or sister is 2–3 times the risk to women without an affected mother or sister.

These epidemiologic studies of familial clustering of breast cancer reveal several findings of practical importance for patient counseling.

1) Close relatives (mothers, sisters and daughters) of breast cancer patients

are at higher risk than more distant relatives. For example, very complete genealogical and tumor registry records in Iceland permitted comparison of risks to various relatives of patients, after adjusting for differing ages and decades of birth of the relatives. Sisters of breast cancer patients were at 3-fold increased risk, patients' mothers at 2-fold increased risk, aunts at 1.6-fold increased risk, but grandmothers and cousins at no increased risk (Tulinius et al, 1982).

2) In populations from various countries, maternal and paternal female relatives have similar risks. That is, there is no evidence that susceptibility is more likely to be passed through the maternal than paternal line. Obviously, mothers are more likely to be affected than fathers, but maternal and paternal aunts, or maternal and paternal grandmothers, have similar risks.

3) Women with both an affected mother and an affected sister are at greater risk than women with either an affected mother or sister. A recent American study surveyed over 1100 nurses who had developed breast cancer and 11 000 nurses without the disease (Bain et al, 1980). Women with either a mother or a sister with breast cancer were at 2-fold greater risk than women with no affected relatives. The few women with affected mothers and sisters were at 5.6-fold greater risk than women with no affected relatives. Similar differences in risk appeared among women who were followed for 5 years as participants in the US Breast Cancer Detection Demonstration Project (Brinton et al, 1982).

4) Daughters of patients are at about the same risk as sisters of patients, once differences in age are taken into consideration (Tulinius et al, 1982; Anderson 1982).

5) Familial breast cancer patients may experience better survival than non-familial patients (Albano et al, 1982; Langlands et al, 1976; Go et al, 1983). These differences appear to be due only in part to earlier diagnosis of familial tumors, or differences in age between familial and nonfamilial patients.

6) The association of tumor histologic type to family history of breast cancer has recently been investigated (Rosen et al, 1982). Sisters of patients with lobular carcinoma were at slightly higher risk than sisters of other patients, whereas sisters of patients with medullary carcinoma were at lower risk. On the other hand, patients with medullary carcinoma were more likely to have affected mothers than were other patients. These medullary carcinoma patients were also younger than other patients. The relationship of histologic type, patients' ages at diagnosis, their relatives' ages, and familial risk is complex and not yet fully understood. Rosen et al conclude that 'no single histologic type of carcinoma was consistently linked to a disproportionately high or low frequency of carcinoma in all classes of relatives.'

7) Familial breast cancer often appears to be strikingly associated with early age at diagnosis and with bilaterality of the tumors. In particular, several studies have shown that familial cases were younger at diagnosis than nonfamilial cases (Langlands et al, 1976; Albano et al, 1982; and review in Petrakis et al, 1982). Similarly, mothers and sisters of women diagnosed at young ages were at greater risk than relatives of women diagnosed at later ages (Bain et al, 1980; Brinton et al, 1982; Ottman et al, 1983). Several studies also have

shown that a higher proportion of familial than nonfamilial cases had bilateral breast cancer (Sakamoto et al, 1978); or that the risks of breast cancer to women with an affected relative were greater if the relative had bilateral rather then unilateral breast cancer (Ottman et al 1983). However, studies in Japan, Sweden, Iceland, and of the women older than 35 years in the American screening program have shown little or no association between age at diagnosis and familiality (Murata et al, 1982; Adami et al, 1981; Tulinius et al, 1982; Brinton et al, 1982). Furthermore, neither the Swedish cohort nor the American screening population demonstrated an association between familial risk and unilateral versus bilateral breast cancer (Adami et al, 1981; Brinton et al; 1982). In the American cohort, the association between bilaterality and increased risk may appear as the population is followed for more than 5 years. Because some studies have shown associations between familial risk, age at diagnosis, and unilateral versus bilateral disease, and others have not, it is important to be careful in applying familial risk estimates derived from one population to women from a different population. The different findings reported in various populations may reflect different reasons for, or manifestations of, familial breast cancer in different populations.

Given the complex epidemiology of familial breast cancer, how can the clinician best advise a patient of her risk? We recently attempted to address this issue in a practical way for patients with different ages at diagnosis and tumor laterality (Ottman et al, 1983). The motivation for this analysis was our observation that epidemiologic results are of little clinical use unless specific estimates of risk at particular times in women's lives are available. We used life table analysis to estimate the cumulative risk of breast cancer to various ages for sisters of breast cancer patients in a population-based series (Table 7.1). These cumulative risk estimates were then used to derive sisters' probability of breast cancer diagnosis within each decade between ages 20 and 70, according to age of diagnosis in the patient and whether the disease was unilateral or bilateral (Table 7.2). These estimates can be used for counselling women with family histories of breast cancer about their risks.

Table 7.1 shows the cumulative probability of breast cancer developing in sisters at different ages. Sisters of patients with bilateral disease had higher risk than sisters of patients with unilateral disease. Among patients with unilateral breast cancer, risks were no higher for sisters of premenopausal patients than for sisters of postmenopausal patients.

Table 7.2 shows the risks of breast cancer within different age-ranges for sisters. Sisters of postmenopausal patients with unilateral disease experienced most of their lifetime risk after age 50. That is, sisters of postmenopausal patients with unilateral disease had much lower risks between ages 30 and 50 (5%) than between ages 50 and 70 (14%). On the other hand, sisters of unilateral premenopausal patients had similar low risk before and after age 50 (5% and 3%, respectively). Risks for sisters of premenopausal patients with bilateral disease were high before age 50 (12%), but after age 50 they were even more alarming (44%).

Relatives of patients with bilateral breast cancer diagnosed at age 40 or younger have by far the greatest risk. However, among sisters of patients with

Table 7.1 Cumulative incidence of breast cancer (in percent) to various ages among sisters of breast cancer patients. Estimates are ranges of two standard errors. Patients (not sisters) are classified by age at diagnosis and tumor laterality.

Tumour laterality and age of diagnosis of patient	Age of sister at end of interval				
	30	40	50	60	70
Bilateral tumors					
Dx ≤ 40 years	0–6	5–17	15–38	23–50	50*
Dx age 41–50	0	2–8	5–13	21–43	21–43
Total ≤ 50 years	0–2	4–10	9–17	31–50	40–50*
Unilateral tumors					
Dx ≤ 40 years	0	0–7	3–14	3–14	2–14
Dx age 41–50	0	0	2–7	3–11	3–11
Total ≤ 50 years	0	0–1	3–7	4–11	4–11
Dx after age 50	0	0	3–8	6–13	9–28
All unilateral patients	0	0–1	4–7	6–12	9–26

* For diseases with completely genetic etiologies, risks to relatives do not exceed 50%. Thus 50% is the biologically reasonable upper estimate for very high risk families. In our sample, the only elderly sister of a young bilateral patient developed breast cancer, so the incidence in our small series was actually higher than 50%.

Table 7.2 Risk of breast cancer (in percent) within given age-ranges for sisters of breast cancer patients. Patients (not sisters) are classified by age at diagnosis and tumor laterality.

Sisters age interval		Diagnosis in patients						Unilateral postmenopausal (≥51)
		Bilateral premenopausal			Unilateral premenopausal			
Beginning	End	(≤40)*	(41–50)	Total	(≤40)	(41–50)	Total	
30	40	8	5	6	4	0	1	0
	50	24	9	12	8	4	5	5
	60	50**	31	39	8	7	7	9
	70	50**	31	50	8	7	7	18
40	50	17	4	7	4	4	4	5
	60	50**	27	35	4	7	7	9
	70	50**	27	48	4	7	7	18
50	60	47	24	30	—	3	3	4
	70	50**	24	44	—	3	3	14
60	70	50**	—	21	—	—	—	10

* Age at diagnosis of patients
** See footnote to Table 7.1

unilateral breast cancer, our data did not confirm the pattern originally described by Anderson (1982) of higher risk for relatives of premenopausal patients than for relatives of postmenopausal patients. Although sisters of breast cancer patients diagnosed before age 40 had higher risk than had sisters of patients diagnosed between ages 41 and 50, the risk to sisters in this second group was no higher than risk to sisters of unilateral postmenopausal patients.

Shortly after we developed the risk estimates in Tables 7.1 and 7.2, Anderson estimated probabilities of breast cancer developing in sisters of familial breast cancer patients, using the same methods (Anderson & Badzioch, 1984). The figures derived from his data on familial breast cancer were lower than ours for sisters of bilateral premenopausal patients and higher than ours for sisters of unilateral premenopausal patients. These differences underscore the need for caution in applying probability estimates for counseling. Some of the risks to sisters in our sample were surprisingly high. These high probabilities resulted in part from small numbers in some of the age intervals, leading to wide standard errors of the risk estimates (see Table 1). For diseases with simple genetic etiologies, risks to relatives do not exceed 50%, so 50% is a realistic upper risk estimate based on biological considerations. However, risk estimates based on families known to be at high risk can lead to artifically low or high estimates. In Anderson's series, risk estimates are actually artificially low, because he 'overcorrected' for the way in which families were ascertained. That is, his patients were selected by identifying breast cancer patients whose medical records reported a positive family history. Relatives reported in the medical record to be affected were excluded from the risk estimation (Anderson 1972). Therefore, if a woman's medical record listed her sister as having breast cancer, the sister was excluded. This procedure is likely to underestimate risk to sisters of breast cancer patients, because many of the sisters with breast cancer will have been listed in the records and thus excluded from the calculations. In addition, risk estimates based on women with *three* relatives with breast cancer (the index case and her two affected relatives) may be inappropriate for counselling women with only one relative affected.

There remains substantial heterogeneity in risk for breast cancer among relatives of different patients, even within our diagnostic classes. Families vary in their susceptibility to breast cancer. Differences in risk among relatives of patients in various diagnostic classes probably result from differences in the proportion of patients belonging to families with extremely high risk. Thus the high risk among relatives of patients with bilateral breast cancer diagnosed before age 40 probably occurs because a large proportion of these patients belong to families with unusually high susceptibility. This also means that some women are not at increased risk, despite diagnosis of bilateral disease at an early age in one of their relatives.

The estimates in Tables 7.1 and 7.2 are useful for counseling women about the risks for breast cancer associated with family histories of various types, but the standard errors of these estimates estimates are large. Nonetheless, these estimates do give some indication of the probability of a woman being affected by breast cancer. Women with family histories of breast cancer often believe their risks to be far higher than those we have reported. Thus, even a risk estimate as high as 50% may be reassuring to a woman who believes she is certain to get breast cancer. However, a woman's age and whether her disease is unilateral or bilateral are only partial indications of the risk of breast cancer for her relatives. It is also important to determine how many relatives in the family have had breast cancer, and the genetic relation of the affected relatives to the woman at risk. Assessment of risk of breast cancer should thus be based on family history, on the characteristics of breast cancer in affected relatives, and on epidemiological characteristics such as the woman's age and age at first pregnancy. Until there is a direct way of assessing risk of breast cancer for individuals, one of the most important areas for breast cancer research is the search for genetic, endoctrine, and/or immunological markers that distinguish high-risk from lower-risk women.

Genetic studies of familial breast cancer: patterns of inheritance

Because breast cancer clusters in families more frequently than expected by chance, determining the reason for that clustering can contribute both to the understanding of breast cancer etiology and to its control. Three general mechanisms may explain familial clustering: a gene or genes increasing susceptibility to breast cancer may be biologically inherited, behaviours or life styles increasing susceptibility may be culturally inherited, or related individuals may be exposed together to environmental or infectious disease agents. These mechanisms are not mutually exclusive and may act in concert to produce familial disease. A variety of study designs and analytic methods have been devised to disentangle these alternative possibilities. For the study of breast cancer, the most fruitful approach has been the analysis of large pedigrees (Elston, 1980; Go et al, 1983; King et al, 1983). Pedigree analysis allows us to assess whether breast cancer in a family or families occurs in a pattern consistent with Mendelian (or genetic) inheritance of genes greatly increasing susceptibility to the disease. Such models actually test for vertical transmission of breast cancer in families. Consistency of a genetic model for inheritance of breast cancer susceptibility would not preclude cultural or environmental mechanisms for the inheritance of cancer susceptibility (King et al, 1984).

Behavioral factors associated with risk to specific cancers may also be culturally transmitted from parents to their children. Cultural inheritance can, and frequently does, mimic genetic inheritance. For example, families with many cases of lung cancer may occur, not only because of genetic susceptibility, but because the smoking habit is passed from parents to children. In other words, smoking and therefore susceptibility to lung cancer is culturally inherited in such families (Tokuhata & Lilienfeld, 1963; Osann, 1983). Though we know of no cultural influence of comparable importance for breast cancer, it was nevertheless necessary to test such genetic models in those families in which the pattern of breast cancer is consistent with Mendelian inheritance.

The first goal of pedigree analysis is to determine whether a single gene may have a major influence on breast cancer susceptibility. Such susceptibility genes are alleles of DNA sequences of generally normal function. Using pedigree analysis, we can determine how such a hypothetical susceptibility allele is inherited in a Mendelian manner in high-risk families: whether it is dominant or recessive, and whether X-linked (on the X chromosome) or autosomal (on a chromosome other than X or Y). This approach is also referred to as segregation analysis because it specifies how susceptibility segregates in families. In order to determine the mode of Mendelian inheritance of a susceptibility allele, it is not necessary to understand the mode of inheritance often contributes to the ultimate elucidation of the complete biochemical and physiological pathway of disease susceptibility. By delineating the mode of inheritance, pedigree analysis contributes directly to risk assessment and genetic counselling for patients and their relatives.

Alternative modes of inheritance of a susceptibility allele yield different disease for various classes of relatives, such as patients' sisters, mothers, and daughters. By comparing observed disease incidence in each relative class with that expected based on alternative genetic models, it is possible to test various genetic hypotheses (Chapter 4 in Emery, 1976). For example, if susceptibility is inherited as an autosomal dominant allele, sisters and daughters of patients have the same 50% risk of inheriting susceptibility (though not necessarily of being affected), and every case will have at least one susceptible parent. Obviously, if the susceptible parent is the father, the disease is unlikely to be expressed, but susceptibility could still be transmitted.

On the other hand, if susceptibility is inherited as an autosomal recessive allele, patients' sisters are at much higher risk than patients' daughters, because daughters will be susceptible only if the patient mates with someone else carrying at least one copy of the susceptibility allele. In this instance, sisters each have a 25% chance of inheriting susceptibility, whereas the risk to daughters depends on the much lower frequency of the recessive susceptibility allele in the population. If susceptibility is recessive, both parents of a case are usually not susceptible; in fact, there may be little or no history of breast cancer in the extended family. Furthermore, diseases with recessive genetic susceptibility are generally more common in inbred populations in which they occur at all. Sickle cell anemia and cystic fibrosis are examples of diseases with simple recessive inheritance. If breast cancer susceptibility were strongly influenced by an allele with incomplete dominance, susceptibility of patients' sisters, daughters, and mothers would fall between these extreme cases.

For any disease, if susceptibility is X-linked, risks to males and females differ dramatically. For X-linked dominant diseases, risks to females are about twice risks to males, all daughters and no sons of male cases are susceptible, all children of female cases have the same 50% risk of inheriting the susceptibility gene, and every case has at least one susceptible parent. No common diseases are known to have inherited dominant X-linked susceptibility. This mode of inheritance of susceptibility is particularly difficult to evaluate for breast cancer, since males are almost never affected. Thus, a breast cancer patient inheriting susceptibility from an affected paternal grandmother and paternal aunts could be from a family with autosomal dominant susceptibility or X-linked dominant susceptibility. Breast cancer patients separated by at least two generations of males (i.e. affected paternal great-grandmother and great-granddaughter) are stronger evidence for autosomal, rather than X-linked, susceptibility. Recessive X-linked inheritance is highly unlikely for breast cancer because female cases of X-linked recessive disorders almost never occur. The frequency of an X-linked recessive susceptibility gene would have to be unreasonably high to explain breast cancer patterns in high risk families.

For some diseases, the mode of inheritance is clear from the family pedigrees of cases. However, for breast cancer, delineating the mode of inheritance is trickier. Several clinical and epidemiologic characteristics of breast cancer complicate segregation analysis.

1) Breast cancer is almost certainly genetically heterogeneous, so that families are analyzed together that actually have different susceptibility genes. This peril can be avoided by studying individual, very large, extended families, within any one of which it is reasonable to assume only one form of genetic susceptibility appears (Elston, 1980).

2) Breast cancer families are often selected for study in such a way that one or another genetic model is more likely to fit the data. Most commonly, ascertainment bias results from selection of families with many cases of breast cancer, or from including families of every patient in a clinical series. Adjustment for mode of ascertainment is possible in analysis, and a major portion of segregation analysis theory is devoted to working out methods for doing so (Morton, 1982).

3) Not all susceptible people develop breast cancer. Men almost never do, even if they carry a susceptibility gene, and some susceptible women remain unaffected as well. Thus, lifetime risk among female relatives based on incidence data may be considerably lower than that expected based on modes of inheritance of susceptibility alleles. Such 'incomplete penetrance' of susceptibility genes may be due to modifying environmental influences, to influences of other susceptibility genes, and, of course, to normal genetic differences between men and women.

4) Among susceptible women who ultimately develop the disease, age at onset may differ considerably. Thus, at any one time, we know only the disease-free years of an unaffected woman, the distribution of ages at diagnosis of affected women, and the relationships of these women to one another. We need to estimate, for each genetic hypothesis

(a) The probability that a woman is susceptible given her age and current disease status
(b) The remaining lifetime breast cancer risk for susceptible individuals
(c) The goodness of fit of the genetic model.

5) Some cases of breast cancer may occur for entirely environmental reasons even in a family with genetic susceptibility. Because genetic and nongenetic cases of breast cancer may be indistinguishable clinically, both may mistakenly be included as genetic cases, weakening the apparent fit of a genetic model.

These complexities preclude direct application of principles of formal genetics to pedigree analysis of breast cancer in families. Statistical methods for testing genetic hypotheses given these complications have been developed (Elston, 1980; Morton, 1982). For breast cancer, we have tested specific genetic hypothesis against a hypothesis which postulates high disease risk in the absence of inheritance of susceptibility alleles. In each case, tests were also made for an environmental hypothesis, which postulates equal age-specific risk for all women in the same generation, regardless of the disease status of their ancestors (Go et al, 1983). For 16 pedigrees, results were consistent with the hypothesis that breast cancer had a genetic etiology. For two other families, breast cancer appeared more likely to be environmental in origin. Hypotheses postulating three different autosomal dominant susceptibility alleles best explained breast cancer susceptibility in three distinct groups of families:

(1) Families with primarily premenopausal breast cancer and ovarian cancer
(2) Families with primarily postmenopausal breast cancer
(3) Families with breast cancer, brain tumors, sarcoma, leukemia, and adreno-cortical carcinoma in children and young adults.

Age-specific risks of breast cancer among women predicted to be genetically susceptible varied considerably among the three groups of families. Clearly, inherited susceptibility to breast cancer may be used by different genes in different families. Table 7.3 indicates the predicted risk of breast cancer to genetically susceptible women in families with primarily premenopausal breast cancer and ovarian cancer. Women in the same families who do not carry the susceptibility gene are *not* at increased risk.

Table 7.3 Predicted risk of breast cancer to genetically susceptible women in families with primarily premenopausal breast cancer. Risks to American white women in the Third National Cancer Survey are given for comparison. Women in high-risk families who do *not* carry the susceptibility allele are at the low risk of the TNCS women. Predicted risks for women in high risk families with other genetic patterns will be different than those indicated here. See page 90 (From Go et al, 1983)

Age in years	Age-specific risk of breast cancer/1000 women	
	Genetically susceptible women (predicted by model)	TNCS white women
20–24	1.6	0.01
25–29	6.6	0.09
30–34	15	0.23
35–39	23	0.53
40–44	26	1.04
45–49	27	1.59
50–54	22	1.72
55–59	19	1.92
60–64	13	2.26
65–69	9.4	2.34
70–74	6.2	2.60
75–79	4.0	2.95
80–84	2.4	3.01
≥ 85	1.6	3.08

An effective means of verifying a model of genetic transmission of breast cancer susceptibility is through linkage analysis (King, 1982; Chapter 3 in Vogel & Motulsky, 1979). The principle of linkage analysis is that if a hypothetical allele influencing disease susceptibility exists, then it must be a length of DNA on one of the 23 pairs of human chromosomes. If the chromosomal location of the susceptibility allele can be determined, then the susceptibility allele exists, even if its protein product remains unknown. In order to map the chromosomal location of a hypothetical susceptibility gene, 'marker' genes, generally with known chromosomal locations, are used to track the inheritance of each of the 23 autosomes and the X and Y chromosomes through a family. If one allele of one of these marker genes is consistently inherited with disease within a family, then a susceptibility allele may be chromosomally linked to that marker gene in that family. If different genes are responsible for disease susceptibility in different families, those genes could be on different chromosomes. Such genetic heterogeneity can also be confirmed by linkage analysis.

Because segregation analysis indicates that breast cancer susceptibility may be inherited as single genes in some families, linkage of those hypothetical susceptibility genes and each of many marker genes can be evaluated statistically. We compare the odds that breast cancer susceptibility and a specific marker gene are inherited together by chance (in the absence of linkage) with the odds that breast cancer susceptibility and the marker gene are coinherited more often because they are close together on the same chromosome. However, linkage between a susceptibility gene and marker gene does not imply that any particular genotype at the marker gene will be associated with disease susceptibility in the general population, or even among a group of high-risk families. The marker gene simply serves to indicate the general chromosomal location of the susceptibility gene.

The usefulness of linkage analysis depends not only on the power and efficiency of the statistical techniques employed, but also on the number of genetic markers available for analysis. That is, even if a disease susceptibility allele is segregating in a family, it is only possible to demonstrate linkage to a marker locus if an informative genetic marker happens to be on the same chromosome as the susceptibility gene, and to be reasonably close to it. A great many marker would be required to 'cover' the 23 chromosomes. While the human genome is by no means completely covered by markers at present, a great deal of progress is now being made in revealing and mapping genetic markers at the level of DNA rather than proteins (Human Gene Mapping, 1984). The enormous amount of genetic information that can be used for linkage analysis based on DNA markers will enable us within the next few years to map susceptibility genes for any disease for which they exist and for which enough informative families are available. Despite the limited number of markers historically available, linkage analysis has helped elucidate the mode of inheritance of several diseases including breast cancer.

Our linkage analysis of breast cancer susceptibility in the families with primarily premenopausal breast cancer and ovarian cancer indicated that a dominant susceptibility gene predisposing to breast cancer and (in five families) ovarian cancer may be linked to the chromosome 16 marker gene glutamate-pyruvate transaminae, or GPT (King et al, 1983). The odds in favor of this linkage are about 90 to one, which is not sufficiently significant for complete confirmation, given the number of markers tested, but does support the genetic hypothesis for susceptibility to breast cancer in those families. The genetic heterogeneity of the inherited susceptibility to breast cancer was indicated by the fact that GPT was not linked to disease in other families, in which susceptability differed epidemiologically and genetically (King et al, 1983; Cleton et al, 1983). The GPT genotype is not associated with breast cancer risk in the general population, so GPT linkage cannot be used as screening test for breast cancer.

The next steps in the genetic analysis of breast cancer in families will include testing possible linkages in additional families, increasing the information available from these families by development of methods to detect other polymorphic protein and DNA markers and more alleles at existing markers, and continuing to follow high-risk families as new cases of breast cancer appear and other women grow older without developing the disease. GPT has been assigned to the short arm of chromosome 16, also the probable location of genes for a regulator of interferon production and a regulator of antiviral state (Human Gene Mapping, 1984). It would be interesting to investigate linkage between these loci and familial breast cancer.

Elucidation of genetic models for inheritance of susceptibility to breast cancer would have several important implications for breast cancer etiology and prevention. First, it would be possible to detect genetically susceptible young women in families at high risk of breast cancer long before clinical symptoms of the disease appear. Genetic and preventive medical counselling for such individuals would thus become a real possibility. Furthermore, it would be possible to determine how many genetically influenced forms of breast cancer exist, and their patterns of transmission in famillies. It would also be possible to investigate why some genetically susceptible women do not develop breast cancer. The influence of cultural and environmental factors on breast cancer risk in the general population is well established. Do these same factors modify the increased risk of genetically susceptible women, or do other factors, perhaps of less importance in the general population, protect some genetically susceptible women from development of breast cancer (Brinton et al, 1982)?

Finally, what are the biochemical and physiological mechanisms by which a gene increases breast cancer susceptibility? The linkage of a marker locus and breast cancer susceptibility in some families may offer an excellent opportunity to elucidate breast cancer etiology. With the use of linkage analysis, it may be possible to identify genetically susceptible young women who have not yet developed breast cancer and other young women in the same family who are at low risk. By the comparison of appropriate immunologic, biochemical, and endocrinologic parameters of these high- and low-risk young women, it may be possible to determine how breast cancer susceptibility genes are expressed. Such understanding could lead ultimately to the prevention of familial breast cancer.

REFERENCES

Adami H O, Hansen J, Jung B, Rimsten A 1980 Familiality in breast cancer: a case-control study in a Swedish population. British Journal of Cancer 42: 71–77
Adami H O, Hansen J, Jung B, Rimsten A 1981 Characteristics of familial breast cancer in Sweden: absence of relation to age and unilateral versus bilateral disease. Cancer 48: 1688–95
Albano W A, Recabaren J A, Lynch H T, Campbell A S, Maillard J A et al 1982 Natural history of hereditary cancer of the breast and colon. Cancer 50: 360–63
Anderson, D E 1972 A genetic study of human breast cancer. Journal of the National Cancer Institute 48: 1029–34
Anderson D E 1982 Familial predisposition. In: Schottenfeld D, Fraumeni J F (eds) Cancer Epidemiology and prevention. Saunders, Philadelphia p 483–93
Anderson D E, Badzioch M 1984 Risk of familial breast cancer Lancet Feb 18, p 392
Bain C, Speizer F E, Rosner B, Belanger C, Hennekens C H 1980 Family history of breast cancer as a risk indicator for the disease. American Journal of Epidemiology 111: 301–08

Bishop J M 1983 Cancer genes come of age. Cell 32: 1018–20

Brinton L A, Hoover R, Fraumeni J F Jr 1982 Interaction of familial and hormonal risk factors for breast cancer. Journal of the National Cancer Institute. 69: 817–22

Brinton L A, Hoover R, Fraumeni J F Jr 1983 Epidemiology of minimal breast cancer. Journal of the American Medical Association 249: 483–87

Cleton F J, de-Jong-Bakker M, King M C 1983 Genetic analysis of breast cancer in Dutch families: preliminary results. European Organisation for the Research and Treatment of Cancer II:11

Elston R C 1980 Segregation Analysis Advances in Human Genetics 11: 60–121

Emery A E H 1976 Methodology in Medical Genetics. Churchill Livingstone, New York p 157

Go R C P, King M C, Bailey-Wilson J, Elston R C, Lynch H T 1983 Genetic epidemiology of breast cancer and associated cancers in families. I. Segregation analysis. Journal of the National Cancer Institute 71: 455–61

Human Gene Mapping, 7. 1984 Gytogenet. Cell Genetics 37; nos. 1–4

King M C 1982 Genetic and epidemiological analysis of cancer in families: Breast cancer as an example. Cancer Surveys 1: 33–46

King M C, Go R C P. Lynch H T, Elson R C, Terasaki P I et al 1983 Genetic epidemiology of breast cancer and associated cancers in high-risk families. II. Linkage analysis. Journal of the National Cancer Institute 71: 463–67

King M C, Lee G T, Spinner N R, Thomson G, Wrensch M C 1984. Genetic Epidemiology. Annual Reviews of Public Health 5: 1–52

Langlands A O, Kerr G R, Bloomer S M 1976 Familial breast cancer. Clinical Oncology 2: 41–45

Lynch H T, Fain P R, Golgar D, Albano W A, Maillard J A et al 1981 Familial breast cancer and its recognition in an oncology clinic. Cancer 47: 2730–39

Morton N E 1982 Outline of Genetic Epidemiology. Karger, New York p 252

Murata M, Kuno K, Fukami A, Sakamoto G 1982 Epidemiology of familial predisposition for breast cancer in Japan Journal of the National Cancer Institute 69: 1229–34

Osann K 1983 Epidemiology of lung cancer in women. PhD dissertation. U California, Berkeley

Ottman R, Pike M C, King M C, Henderson B E 1983 Estimating risk for familial breast cancer: a practical guide. Lancet: Sept 3, p 556–58

Petrakis N L, Ernster V L, King M C 1982 Breast In: Schottenfeld D, Fraumeni J F (eds) Cancer epidemiology and prevention. Saunders, Philadelphia p. 855–870

Rosen P P, Lesser M L, Senie R T, Kinne D W 1982 Epidemiology of Breast Carcinoma III. Relationship of family history to tumour type. Cancer 50: 171–79

Ruddle F H 1981 A new era in mammalian gene mapping: somatic cell genetics and recombinant DNA methodologies. Nature 294: 115–20

Sakamoto G, Sugano H, Kasumi F 1978 Bilateral breast cancer and familial aggregations. Preventative Medical 7: 225–29

Schimke R N 1978 Genetics and Cancer In Man. Churchill Livingstone, New York p 108

Schottenfeld D, Fraumeni J F (eds) 1982 Cancer Epidemiology and Prevention. Saunders, Philadelphia p 1173

Tokuhata G K, Lilienfeld A M 1963 Familial aggregation of lung cancer in humans. Journal of the National Cancer Institute 30: 289–312

Tulinius H, Day N E, Bjarnason O, Geirsson G, Johannesson G et al 1982 Familial breast cancer in Iceland. International Journal of Cancer 29: 365–71

Vogel F, Motulsky A G 1979 Human Genetics: Problems and Approaches Springer-Verlag, New York p 700

Yunis J J 1983 The chromosomal basis of human neoplasia. Science 221: 227–36

Yuspa S H, Harris C C 1982 Molecular and cellular basis of chemical carcinogenesis. In: Schottenfeld D, Fraumeni J F Cancer epidemiology and prevention. Saunders, Philadelphia p 23–43

8

The history of breast cancer

MICHAEL BAUM

Introduction

To most medical students the history of medicine appears to be an irrelevant study, at best occupying an entertaining hour when listening to a visiting professor lecture, or alternatively seen as a harmless occupation for retired and lonely physicians to end their days tottering under the dusty weight of ancient tracts between the most remote book store rooms and their soft-lit, leather-topped desks. Each generation of students feels that anything written over 20 years ago is of no value for passing examinations and absolutely nothing to do with how they treat patients on the wards. It is the purpose of this chapter to demonstrate just how wrong and even potentially dangerous this attitude may be. To paraphrase Santayana's immortal words: if we are not prepared to learn our lessons from the past we are almost certainly cursed to repeat our mistakes in the future. History is a continuum and our generation is merely a point along this line. What a conceit it is to think for one moment that we are approximating to a true understanding of the subject covered by this book and that our favoured treatments are based on concepts that will stand the test of time.

The history of any science can be described as the elaboration of hypotheses their testing and ultimate refutations followed by conceptual revolutions; further hypothesis building and further refutations: always an approximation towards a truth but never an arrival. The history of breast cancer is the same— the generation of conceptual frameworks followed by 'logical' treatments designed to satisfy the concept, conceptual shifts followed by therapeutic revolutions and so on. Sometimes our concepts have suggested therapeutic nihilism, whilst at other points in the history of our subject, conceptual rationalization has demanded mutilations and noxious remedies that have increased the sum of suffering of countless trusting and hapless women.

The object of this chapter therefore is to trace the development and rejection of theories concerning the nature of breast cancer, together with the evolution and abandonment of treatments designed to satisfy the needs of the dominant theory of the day.

The ancient world

If thou examinest a man (person) having bulging tumours of his breast and thou findest that swellings have spread over his breast; if thou puttest thy hand upon his breast upon these tumours, and thou findest them very cool, there being no fever at all herein when thy hand touches him; they have no granulations, they form no fluid, they do not generate secretions of fluid and they are bulging to thy hand. Thou shouldst say concerning him. There is no treatment.

This translation of the Edwin Smith Surgical Papyrus by J. H. Breasted was published in 1930. Many scholars have suggested that this is evidence that the ancient Egyptians distinguished inflammatory mastitis from carcinoma of the breast. I would go further and suggest that this passage described locally advanced breast cancer perhaps with satellite nodules and demonstrates the wisdom of the ancient and anonymous author in recognizing the futility of any intervention. This therapeutic nihilism must have resulted from the accumulated experience in vainly trying to influence the natural history of the advanced disease.

In or around 400 BC, Hippocrates went even further when he wrote 'It is better to give no treatment in cases of hidden cancer (referring to non-ulcerating breast cancer); treatment causes speedy death, but to omit treatment is to prolong life' (Hippocrates, 1953). Hippocrates went on to develop his ideas concerning the natural humours of the body and to suggest that cancer like most other disease processes resulted from an imbalance of these humours, but as far as I can judge he never described how these humoral imbalances could be corrected to the advantage of patients with breast cancer. Approximately 500 years later, during the flowering of the Greco/Roman period of medicine, Celsus made probably the first attempt to describe, classify and stage carcinoma of the breast. He suggested four stages (1) Early malignancy (2) Cancer without ulcer (3) Ulcerating cancer and (4) Fungating cancer. In contrast to the teachings of Hippocrates he felt that treatment was contraindicated in the three late stages but of some value in the earliest stage. (De Moulin, 1983).

In approximately 200 AD, Galen, who studied in Alexandria and practiced in Rome, became the most influential physician of the then known world. He further extended the Hippocratic humoral theory of disease and taught that cancer was related to the accumulation of an excess of black bile (melancholia) that coagulated in the breast. He supported this view by suggesting that women clear themselves of black bile during their monthly periods and therefore after the menopause they are no longer cleansed. This conveniently explained the increasing incidence of breast cancer amongst women in their fifth and sixth decades. If such was the case it would appear logical to cleanse the women again by repeated purgation and bleeding, coupled with diets with putatively low melancholinergic properties. (De Moulin, 1983). This is probably the first and one of the finest examples of what I like to describe as conceptual rationalizations of therapy for breast cancer. Note also that the disease was considered a systemic disorder; but that didn't stop physicians and protosurgeons from using topical applications for ulcers and breast amputation for the smaller tumours. It is a piece of almost black comedy to read how those ancient surgeons hazarding amputation of the breast were encouraged not to stop the bleeding too quickly in order to allow the excess of evil humours to escape.

Such was the charisma of Galen and so rapidly did his teachings become the orthodoxy that for almost 1200 years no-one dared challenge the Galenic doctrine. The dark ages must have been very dark indeed for women with breast cancer apart from the two fortunates who enjoyed miraculous cures of their disease through to ministrations of Saints Kosmas and Damian (The Patron Saints of the Royal College of Surgeons of England). (Heinemann, 1974).

The renaissance

The Renaissance is usually remembered as the rebirth of interest in the arts of ancient Greece; with painting, sculpture and literature throwing off the shackles of the orthodox church, the broadening of study to include liberal subjects and the precious gift of enquiry. This new found freedom of enquiry encouraged developments in anatomy and pathology but at the same time lead to some bizzare and infertile pathways in oncology. For example, Ambrose Paré (1510–1590) the great french military surgeon, advised women against gossip in order to avoid breast cancer (perhaps also a great male chauvinist pig) and recommended treating ulcerated cancer with puppy dogs or kittens freshly split into two with the warm viscera applied to the lesion. (De Moulin, 1983). However, to his credit he did recognize involvement of the homolateral axillary nodes in the disease and advocated the use of ligatures to staunch the bleeding after surgery.

Wilhelm Fabry (1565–1634) also known as Fabricius who practiced in Germany, considered that cancer was caused by milk curdling in the breast and is thought to have performed the first axillary node dissection via a counter incision (De Moulin, 1983). (Mastectomy in those days was a simple guillotine amputation with cautery to control the haemorrhage).

Gabrielle Falloppio (1523–62) who was professor of anatomy and surgery at Padua, modified Galen's humoural theory and introduced a non-natural bile which was a combustion product of other humours. He suggested that cancers consisted of a blend of blood and burnt melancholic humour with the degree of malignancy related to the relative proportions of these two substances, with inflammatory carcinoma having the worst prognosis as a result of the most disadvantagenous combination. He was the first to describe pectoral fixation of advanced breast cancer and used this physical sign as evidence of inoperability! (Rather, 1978). Unfortunately he persisted in advising venesection to rid the body of burnt black bile (same treatment, different rationale!).

The 17th and 18th centuries

The start of the 17th Century saw the beginning of the waning influence of the humoural theory of cancer in favour of particular theories of disease due to mechanical defects and hydrodynamic processes. These changes in attitudes were no doubt brought about by Harvey's description of the circulation of the blood in 1628, together with the adoption of the cartesian view of the body as a perfect machine.

Thomas Bartholin (1616–1680) first described the lymphatic system allowing both humoral and mechanical theories of oncogenesis to coexist. The tumours it was suggested, were coagulems of lymph developing proximal to a blockage of lymphatic vessels. (A viewpoint echoed as recently as 1955 by the great English surgeon/pathologist Sampson Handley.) But perhaps the most important development of this period that would in time allow a revolutionary approach to the understanding of cancer was the description of the first microscope by Antoni van Leeuwenhook (1632–1723). This is but one example in the history of science where the invention of an instrument that extended the human powers of observation also extended the human capacity for the generation of hypotheses.

At the same time physicians were arguing about the traumatic psychological and contagious inductions of cancer, whilst still not capable of understanding how the patients died of metastases. For example, Nicholas Tulp (1593–1674) the famous dutch anatomist and surgeon, believed that patients died from auto-intoxication from their ulcerated cancers. (De Moulin, 1983). He was also responsible for the single anecdote that convinced generations of doctors that breast cancer was a contagious disease as a result of being called to treat, both mistress and servant of the same household, for cancer of the breast. Tulp was of course immortalized in Rembrant's painting of 'The Anatomy Lesson'. The artist himself unwittingly contributed to the subject in his hauntingly beautiful painting entitled 'Bathsheba at her toilet.' The model for this work completed in 1655 was Rembrant's mistress Hendrickje Stoffles. Careful examination of the upper outer quadrant of her left breast demonstrates the pathagnomonic dimple of a cancer. She died 9 years after this painting was completed and her mode of dying was suggestive of metastatic breast cancer. (Braithwaite & Shugg, 1983).

In the early 18th century tumours of all sorts were still grouped together with persistence of the ancient distinction between 'scirrhous' and 'carcinomatous' tumours. The former being premalignant and the latter lethaly malignant. The aetiology of the disease was still considered a combination of local and systemic causes. The local causes included trauma, tight clothes and curdled milk, whilst the systemic factors were related to blood components, for example 'yellow bile' from serum; 'Phlegm' from stagnant serum; 'black bile', the clot of extruded red blood cells; 'Materia phlogistica' the component of blood thought to develop into pus. Most physicians favoured the theory that materia phlogistica coagulated internally to produce a scirrhous, although John Hunter (1728–1793) the influential London surgeon favoured the coagulated lymph theory. (Dobson, 1959). John Hunter considered to be the father of British surgical science conducted certain simplistic experiments to support his hypothesis.

Other theories abounded including poisons, acidity, alkalinity, psychological trauma, bad diet and nulliparity. The last three find some support to this day.

But perhaps the two most important conceptual advances can be attributed to the French surgeons Le Dran (1685–1770) and Petit (1674–1750) who explained the nature of metastases as either haematogenous or lymphatic spread of the disease to the axilla and distant organs. (Petit, 1774). Unfortunately treatment was still lagging far behind conceptual advances with guillotine amputation in rare selected cases of early disease and disgusting topical applications, diet, purgation and bleeding for most other cases. However, for the first time we can see the prodromal symptoms of the current controversy of conservative versus radical surgery with William Cheseldon of St. Georges Hospital London (1688–1752) advocating lumpectomy and Louis Petit of Paris advocating the more radical approach. (De Moulin, 1983). Ironically the London/Paris position appears to have become reversed over the last 200 years.

The 19th century

The Cook and Housekeeper's complete and universal dictionary complied by Mrs. Mary Eaton at the beginning of the 19th century describes the popular management of cancer, slotted between canaries and candied angelica. (Eaton, 1822). Mrs. Eaton suggests that 'this cruel disorder' can be cured in 3 days by a simple application without the need of surgery. The topical agent was made from dough mixed with hogs lard applied to the affected part spread on a piece of white leather. 'This, if it do no good is perfectly harmless, several persons have derived great benefit from this application and it has seldom been known to fail'.

It would be reasonable to judge from this kind of evidence that many of the poor and simple folk of this era were fortunate enough to avoid the unwelcome attentions of the medical establishment treating themselves with harmless remedies whilst their cancers ran their natural course. At the same time the medical establishment were asking themselves some very pertinent questions about the nature of cancer. In 1802 a meeting took place in Edinburgh present at which were John Abernethy, John Hunter's pupil and his successor as Surgeon at St. Bartholomew's Hospital, Mathew Baillie a nephew of Hunter's and the author of 'Morbid Anatomy', Robert Willen, founder of British dermatology and John Hunter's brother-in-law, Everand. This committee discussed the question 'May cancer be regarded at any period or under any circumstances merely as a local disease, or does the existence of cancer in one part afford a presumption that there is a tendency to a familiar alteration in other parts of the animal?' The result of their deliberations was published in July 1806 in the Edinburgh Medical and Surgical Journal (Shimkin, 1957) and to some extent pre-empted the debate that started in the 1950s and continues to rage to this day. Nevertheless, breast cancer was by now treated as a local disease and a beautiful and heartbreaking description of James Syme (Professor of Surgery in Glasgow) performing a mastectomy in 1830, in the absence of any form of anaesthesia, appears in the story 'Rab and his friends' by John Brown. The courageous young woman survived this procedure only to die of septicaemia in the following week. James Syme could hardly be blamed for this in the era before Lister's revolutionary discoveries and is to be credited as first to make the association between involved axillary nodes and a poor prognosis. In 1842 he wrote as follows: 'The result of operations for carcinoma when the glands are affected is almost always unsatisfactory however perfectly they may seem to have been taken away. The reason for this is probably that the glands do not take part in the disease unless the system is strongly disposed to it'. (Syme, 1984).

Improvements in the microscope in the mid 19th century allowed the study of the cellular aspects of cancer and the foundation of cancer histology as a science. This science was blemished by problems with the interpretation of artifacts due to the poor preparation of specimens. It is likely that these artifacts led to the 'Blastema' theory of cancer promoted by Karl Rokitansky (1804–1878) and Sir James Paget (1814–1899). (Paget, 1874). The 'Blastema' was considered to be a primitive form of cell seen as a solid amorphous substance under the microscope (?fibrin) capable of giving rise to cancers at any site within the stroma of healthy organs. This view was attacked by Rudolf Virchow (1821–1902) who suggested that cancers arose from normal cells in reaction to abnormal stimuli, a singularly modern viewpoint, (Virchow, 1863–1873). Yet paradoxically it was Virchow who promoted the view of the centrifugal spread of cancer along the lymphatics by cellular proliferation whilst Sir James Paget believed in a humoral mechanism of metastasis via the blood stream. Virchow's viewpoint became dominant and contributed to the evolution of the radical mastectomy.

The late 19th century and early 20th century

Gross's (1880) treatise on breast cancer provides a clear insight into the natural history of the disease in the immediate pre-Halsted era. He described a series of 616 cases, 70% of whom had skin infiltration on presentation and in 25% of whom the skin was ulcerated; 64% had extensive involvement of axillary nodes and 27% had obvious supraclavicular nodal involvement. As a result of the attitude of that time that the risks of surgery outweighed the benefits offered by such treatment, he considered it ethical to follow the natural course of 97 cases who received nothing other than 'constitutional support'.

From this study he described how skin infiltration appeared, on average, 14 months after a tumour was first detected, ulceration occurred on average 6 months after that, and fixation to the chest wall after a further 2 months. Invasion of the other breast was seen if the patient lived on average 32 months after the lump first appeared. 25% of these untreated cases exhibited obvious distant metastases within 1 year and 25% after 3 years, while 5% of this series died 5 years or more after presentation.

The development of the classical radical mastectomy in the latter part of the nineteenth century may be credited to both Halsted (1898) and Meyer (1894), but it must also be remembered that the operation was designed on the basis of the pathological teachings of Virchow and Samson Handley, which I shall henceforth refer to as the Halsted/Handley hypothesis. It was assumed that a cancer spread in continuity from its origin as columns of malignant cells. These passed along the lymphatic channels until they were arrested temporarily in the first group of regional lymph nodes, which were thought to act as filter traps. It was further assumed that when the filtration capacity of these lymph nodes was exhausted they acted as a nidus for tertiary spread to more distant lymph nodes and then via the fascial planes to the skeleton and the vital organs. Halsted (1907) even went so far as to suggest that there was no skeletal involvement unless there was an overlying cutaneous metastasis with the skeleton being involved as a result of continuity from the original growth via the skin metastasis. Accepting these beliefs it seemed quite reasonable that radical en bloc surgery would cure more patients than local amputation of the breast alone, and for a short period in the early 1920 some surgeons were taking this matter to the logical conclusion and advocating forequarter amputation together with radical clearance of the breast when the disease had spread locally into the upper arm. (Evans, 1923). For that matter, it must be remembered that even such relatively recent developments as the super-radical mastectomy, postoperative radiation after classical mastectomy and any other permutations of local surgery with radiotherapy to the mediastinal and axillary lymph nodes were developed in an attempt to achieve even wider fields of tumour ablation, but even these developments were still based on the blind acceptance of the Halsted/Handley hypothesis, which had become firmly rooted as surgical dogma.

Karl Popper (1959) once wrote that 'instead of discussing the probability of the hypothesis, we should try to assess what test, what trials it has withstood. We should try to assess how far it has been able to prove its fitness to survive'. In retrospect, it is surprising how long the Halsted/Handley hypothesis did survive in the face of such overwhelming evidence against its fitness to do so. First of all there was never any prima facie evidence that the introduction of the classical radical operation did anything to improve the mortality rates from carcinoma of the breast. For example, Gross of Philadelphia (1880) was able to describe a series of patients treated with simple mastectomy alone with a 9% 10 year survival. Lewis and Rinehoff's (1932) classical account of the results from the Johns Hopkins Hospital of patients treated by radical mastectomy between 1898 and 1932 reported only a 12% 10 year survival. There was no doubt that the radical operation reduced the incidence of local recurrence, but in no way improved the survival rates. One can easily ascribe any apparent improvements between the 1930's and today simply representing the better selection of cases for mastectomy, particularly as a result of the work of Haagensen (1971) who defined the grave prognostic signs of locally advanced disease. The second inconsistency with the classical pathological model is that it failed to describe the well-recognized heterogeneity of behaviour of breast cancer commonly encountered in clinical practice. On the one hand, women may present with pathological fractures of the bone or leucoerythroblastic anaemia due to bone marrow involvement, with primary tumours which are undetectable and without lymph node involvement. At the other extreme, some women can survive in excess of 10 years with enormous primary tumours and no treatment.

Surgeons who stubbornly cling to the radical school of thought not only ignore this evidence, but also ignore recent developments in out understanding of tumour biology. For example, it is now known that cancer can gain direct access to the circulation by venous invasion. Furthermore, there a lympho-venous communications which would allow embolizing cancer cells to bypass the lymph nodes. The lymph nodes themselves cannot be considered as effective filters as the cancer cells can traverse them with impunity, as shown by the classical experiments of Bernard Fisher (1970).

The roots of controversy 1950–1970

Macdonald (1951) coined the phrase 'biological predeter-minism' to explain the behaviour of solid tumours in humans. In a closely argued paper he attempted to ridicule the conventional approach to cancer therapy. He postulated that if a period of localized tumour growth is associated with either subjective or objective evidence of its presence, treatment should be able to produce a 100% cure. Therefore, providing that patients are educated to recognize these signs and symptoms, and on recognition proceed to get medical advice without delay, cure rates should continue to improve, eventually to the 100% level. However, in spite of a health education programme in the USA directed at the early diagnosis of cancer, and launched 20 years before Macdonald wrote his paper, the age-adjusted death rates of cancer were increasing rather than decreasing. Furthermore, he presented data which suggested that 'delay' on the part of the patient did not affect the stage at presentation of the tumour; the results of treatment for breast cancer were little different if the patient delayed for 1 month or 12 months.

He concluded therefore that the outcome of treatment is predetermined by the biological nature of the disease:

> This preoccupation with therapeutic seizure of time by its neoplastic forelock rests on the assumption that the cancer is treated more efficiently during the nebulous period when it is yet limited to its site of origin . . . . The wide range of biological potential exhibited by human cancer is determined early in the preclinical phase of the disease—apparently early cancer by historical and dimensional criteria may be biologically late.

Park and Lees (1951) writing in the same year as Macdonald expressed a similar point of view. Starting with the null hypothesis that cancer is incurable until it is proved curable, they postulated that proof is impossible because the natural history of breast cancer is not known. They suggested that there was no 'available time margin' between the time that the tumour reached diagnos-able proportions and its dissemination.

This view was supported by evidence which failed to relate improved survival to short delay by patients. Again their conclusion was that the outcome is predetermined by variations in the growth rate, infiltrative power and metastatic potential of the breast cancer, in addition to its chronological age. But host factors, such as age and general health, may also be important.

McKinnon (1954) took the argument one step forward. He postulated that there might be two types of breast cancer: a metastasizing variety which would be incurable and a non-metastasizing variety which would be curable. The former would present as stages II, III and IV diseases, whilst the latter would present as stage I.

The same theme was taken up again by Devitt (1965). By this time the subject of cancer immunology was developing and the host defence factor could be inserted into the equation of biological predeteriminism. Or, as Devitt succinctly put it: 'Metastases to axillary nodes are an expression of a poor prognosis rather than a determinant'.

More recently Devitt (1976) has reviewed the evidence that 'early' cancers are slow-growing tumours and 'late' cancers are aggressive tumours. He notes that the interval between treatment and recurrence, and that between recurrence and death are longer for those cancers which are diagnosed 'early' than for those diagnosed as 'late'. He concludes that the timing of initial treatment appears to have little influence on the growth behaviour of breast cancer as reflected in survival rates.

However, this conclusion cannot go unchallenged and it would be invidious to ignore the findings of the Screening Program of the New York Health Insurance Plan. This study included 62 000 women of 40–46 years of age, 31 000 of whom were randomly selected and offered screening by clinical examination and mammography on four occasions at annual intervals. The published results indicate that in the screened population breast cancer was detected at an earlier stage and that deaths within seven years of enrolment were reduced by approximately on-third among the women over the age of 50. (Strax et al, 1967). This would seem powerful evidence for the traditional concept of an arithmetic spatial progression related to duration of the disease.

The contemporary or fashionable hypothesis

Within the passage of a decade the Halstedian dogma has been replaced with a fashionable new hypothesis which in its own turn has been translated into a new dogma in many centres of the world. Breast cancer is now considered a systemic disease at the time of presentation with the degree of lymph; node involvement symptomatic of the extent of residual tumour burden following local therapy. Second-order hypotheses suggest that the time and rate of systemic spread depend not only on the innate aggressiveness of the tumour but the immunocompetence of the host. The therapeutic consequences of this paradigm shift has been to minimize the importance of loco/regional therapy and concentrate on systemic approaches directed at the putative micrometastases. Experience with advanced disease has demonstrated something like 30% objective remissions with endocrine therapy against approximately 60% objective remissions with combination cytotoxic chemotherapy.

The third-order hypothesis would suggest therefore that adjuvant chemotherapy following mastectomy should prolong survival in node positive cases. The undoubted short term toxicity of this approach has to be accepted in anticipation of long term benefits. Failure of this approach in clinical trials

(Baum & Berstock, 1982) has been dismissed by many on the basis that the drugs were given too late or in too mall a dose. (Bonnadonna & Valagussa, 1976). We now have a new therapeutic dogma and to repeat what I wrote in the introduction—if we are not prepared to learn our lessons from the past we are almost certainly cursed to repeat our mistakes in the future. The last decades of the 20th Century are part of the continuum of history; in order to be proud of the contributions our generation has made to the understanding and management of breast cancer, let us continue to question all aspects of the fashionable new model of the disease.

One last word concerns the history of the philosophy of science itself. My perspective of the subject I concede has been strongly biased by my Popperian view of the logic of scientific discovery (Popper, 1959). This philosophy has its roots in the teachings of Francis Bacon and Sir Isaac Newton, but has as its unique contribution the acceptance of uncertainty with the journey towards truth an unending quest. In addition, Popper demands that our experiments should be set up to falsify our hypotheses not to have them corroborated. Alternative approaches to the history of science exist as for example Kuhn's (1970) view of the revolutionary scientist whose hypotheses receive spectacular corroboration and in so doing redirect scientific discovery. To my mind these two approaches are easily reconciled explaining both the history and the method of science. (Baum, 1983). At the same time it must be recognized that a popular disenchantment with deductive logic exists finding its most eloquent and persuasive voice in the writings of Fritjof Capra. The metaphysical conceptual shift which has been required to explain recent developments in subatomic nuclear physics has been taken up as the half-baked philosophical justification for 'holistic' medicine. I think they are terribly wrong but as a true scientist I can't be absolutely certain!

Acknowledgements

I wish to thank Professor D.M. Dent of the University of Cape Town for giving me a facsimile of the Edwin Smith Papyrus together with a copy of its translation by J. H. Breasted. I also wish to acknowledge the help of Miss Elizabeth Skinner of the Cancer Research Campaign for finding me the reference from the Cook and Housekeepers Dictionary of 1822. As always I must thank my wife for her tolerance and her typing. Finally, I draw readers attention to the wonderful book on the History of Breast Cancer by Daniel de Moulin (Publishers, Martinus Nyhoff) which was a source of inspiration and directed me to much new and fascinating source material.

REFERENCES

Baum M, Berstock D A 1982 Breast cancer, adjuvant therapy. In: Clinics in Oncology, Breast Cancer. W B Saunders, London. Vol 1, No 3, p 901–916
Baum M 1983 Quack cancer cures or scientific remedies? Clinical Oncology 9:275
Bonnadonna G, Valagussa P 1976 Dose response effect of adjuvant chemotherapy in breast cancer. New England Journal of Medicine 249:405
Braithwaite P A, Shugg D 1983 Rembrandt's Bathsheba: the dark shadow of the left breast. Annals of the Royal College of Surgeons 65:337

Breasted J H 1930 The Edwin Smith Papyrus. University of Chicago Press, Chicago, p 403–406
Clendenning L 1960 Sourcebook of medical history. Dover Publishers, New York, p 346–354
De Moulin D 1983 A short history of cancer. Martinus Nyhoff Publishers, Boston, The Hague, Lancaster
Devitt J E 1965 The significance of regional lymph node metastases in breast carcinoma. Canadian Medical Association Journal 93:289
Devitt J E 1976 Clinical prediction of growth behaviour. In: Stoll B A (ed) Risk factors in breast cancer, Heineman Medical, London, p 110
Dobson J 1959 John Hunter's views on cancer. Annals of the Royal College of Surgeons 1:176
Eaton M 1822 The cook and housekeeper's universal dictionary. L & R Childs, London
Evans W H 1923 The diseases of the breast. University of London Press Ltd, London, p 416
Fisher B 1970 The surgical dilemma in the primary therapy of invasive breast cancer. A critical appraisal. In: Current problems in surgery, Year Book Publishers, Chicago
Gross S W 1880 A practical treatise of tumours of the mammary gland. Appleton, New York
Haagensen C D 1971 Disease of the breast. W B Saunders, Philadelphia
Halsted W S 1898 The radical operation for the cure of carcinoma of the breast. John Hopkins Hospital Reports 28:557
Halsted W S 1907 The results of operations for the cure of cancer of the breast. Annals of Surgery 1:46
Handley W S 1955 The genesis & prevention of cancer. John Murray, London, p 246–247
Heinemann K, Kosmas & Damian 1974 Medical History Journal 9:255
Hippocrates 1953 Nature of Man. In: Jones W H S translation 'Hippocrates' Loeb Classical Library, Wm Heinemann, London, Vol 4
Kuhn T S 1970 The structure of scientific revolutions. Chicago University Press, Chicago
Lewis D, Rinehoff W F 1932 A study of the results of operations for the cure of carcinoma of the breast performed at the Johns Hopkins Hospital for 1889–1931. Annals of Surgery 95:336
MacDonald I 1951 Biological predeterminism in human cancer. Surgery Gynaecology and Obstetrics 92:443
McKinnon N E 1954 Control of cancer mortality. Lancet I 251
Meyer W 1894 The improved method of the radical operation for cancer of the breast. Medical Record 46:746
Paget J 1874 Discussions on cancer. Transactions of the Pathological Society of London 25:287
Park W S, Lees J C 1951 The absolute curability of cancer of the breast. Surgery, Gynaecology and Obstetrics 93:129
Petit J L 1774 (Cited by De Moulin). Oeuvres Posthumes de chirugie, Prault, Paris, Vol 1
Popper K R 1959 The logic of scientific discovery. Hutchinson, London
Rather J L 1978 The genesis of cancer. The Johns Hopkins University Press, Baltimore and London, p 14–19
Shimkin M B 1957 Thirteen questions. Some historical outlines for cancer research. Journal of the National Cancer Institute 19(2):295
Strax P, Venett L, Shapiro S, Gross J 1967 Mammography and clinical examination in mass screening for cancer of the breast. Cancer 20:2184
Syme J 1842 Principles of surgery, Bailliere Tindall, London
Virchow R 1863–1873 (Cited by De Moulin). Die Krankhaften Geschwulste, Hirshwald Publishers, Berlin. Vol 1

9 *The requirement for clinical trials in breast cancer*

RICHARD D. GELBER and ARON
GOLDHIRSCH

Introduction

Clinical trials are widely used to gain information about therapies for patients with cancer. However, adoption of the prospective clinical trial is a fairly recent development. Bull (1959), Mike (1981), and Pocock (1983) summarize some historical perspectives in the development of medical investigations. Prior to the 17th century, physicians applied their own favorite remedies with empirical evaluation of their effectiveness. Hippocrates recommended that 'one must attend in medical practice not primarily to plausible theories, but to experience combined with reason.' In the 17th century, Roger Bacon proposed that more emphasis be placed on experience and that learned physicians contribute information on remedies tried and approved by experiment for the cure of particular diseases. The need for controlled clinical experiments was recognized by some in the 18th century. The British philosopher, George Berkeley, was convinced of the great curing powers of tar-water, prepared by mixing a gallon of water with a quart of tar and removing the supernatant after 3 days. Berkeley proposed that a clinical trial be conducted in which patients were to be 'put into two hospitals at the same time of the year and provided with the same necessities of diet and lodging; and, for further care, let one have a tub of tar-water and an old woman; the other hospital, what attendants and drugs you please.' (Berkeley, 1752).

At about the same time, Lind (1753) planned a comparative trial of the most promising treatments for scurvy. He describes the controlled trial as follows:

> I took 12 patients in the scurvy on board the Salisbury at sea. The cases were as similar as I could have them . . . they lay together in one place . . . and had one diet common to them all. Two of these were ordered a quart of cider a day. Two others took 25 guts of elixir vitriol . . . Two others took two spoonfuls of vinegar . . . Two were put under a course of sea water . . . Two others had each two oranges and one lemon given them each day . . . Two others took the bigness of a nutmeg. The most sudden and visible good effects were perceived from the use of oranges and lemons, one of those who had taken them being at the end of 6 days fit for duty . . . The other . . . was appointed nurse to the rest of the sick.

Both of these studies indicate an awareness for the need to control extraneous or confounding factors in the evaluation of medical therapies. Similar settings and comparable diets were considered to be important aspects of the study design.

It was not until 1834 that the French physician, P. C. A. Louis, elaborated on the use of 'the numerical method' of assessing therapies:

> As to different methods of treatment, if it is possible for us to assure ourselves of the superiority of one or other among them in any disease whatever, having regard to the different circumstances of age, sex and temperament, of strength and weakness, it is doubtless to be done by enquiring if under these circumstances a greater number of individuals have been cured by one means than another. Here again it is necessary to count. And it is, in great part at least, because hitherto this method has been not at all, or rarely employed, that the science of therapeutics is still so uncertain; that when the application of the means placed in our hands is useful we do not know the bounds of this utility.

Dr. Louis also discussed the need for the exact observation of patient outcome, knowledge of the natural progress of untreated controls, precise definition of disease prior to treatment, and careful observation of deviations from intended treatment. Dr. Louis also pointed out, as is the case today, that 'the numerical method . . . offers real difficulties in its execution for, on the one hand, it neither can, nor ought to be applied to any other than exact observations, and these are not common, and on the other hand, this method requires much more labour and time than the most distinguished members of our profession can dedicate to it. But what signifies this reproach, except that the research of truth requires much labour and is beset with difficulties.' The ideas of Dr. Louis on the numerical method and its applications are perhaps even more important today.

Surgical procedures

Due primarily to the discovery of general anesthetics, many advances in surgery were observed during the 19th century. The effectiveness of many of these procedures was so dramatic as to deny the need for control groups and substantial patient numbers. For example, Lister (1870) carried out a study of amputation operations comparing a 43% mortality in 35 cases before the use of antiseptics with a 15% mortality in 40 cases treated by antiseptic procedures. Lister cautioned that 'the numbers are doubtless too small for a satisfactory statistical comparison' which is reality was not true ($\chi^2 = 7.19$, $p < 0.01$). A warning about the possible biases of his retrospective comparison with a historical control group would have been more appropriate as case selection for the operation or other relevant features might have changed over time.

Unfortunately, the informal approach to surgical research continues to dominate the literature today and carries the risk of falsely establishing poor or inadequate surgical procedures as being effective. Even today, arguments are made against conducting controlled trials for evaluating new operations (Bonchek, 1979). The arguments include the fact that surgical procedures exhibit a learning curve phenomenon in which the operative results will improve with repeated practice. The variability of technical skill by surgeon makes the procedure not precisely reproducible and the results uncertain. Furthermore, technical advances in prosthetic devices are being made so rapidly that results from controlled trials of surgical procedures become obsolete soon after they are published.

Historically, breast cancer was treated almost exclusively by surgery alone. The Halsted-Patey hypothesis dictated that the surgery be extensive in order that the spread of the disease (assumed to be mediated exclusively via the lymph node chain) be arrested. This hypothesis was only questioned recently, but has yet to be adequately tested. Veronesi and colleagues (1981) reported the results of a randomized clinical trial comparing radical mastectomy with quadrantectomy, axillary clearance and postsurgical radiotherapy to the partially conserved breast. Patients with positive axillary nodes also received adjuvant chemotherapy. At 3 years of follow-up, the results for the two treatment programs applied to the patients who entered this study were comparable. However, as radiation therapy was an adjuvant to the breast conserving procedure, the belief that radical mastectomy yields the same outcome in terms of control of disease as quadrantectomy and axillary clearance is not justified based on these results. The same problem is encountered in the NSABP study B-04 (Fisher et al 1985b), in which all patients with clinically positive nodes who had total mastectomy were also given adjuvant radiation therapy. Thus, the widespread belief that data exist to show total mastectomy to be as effective as radical mastectomy is based only on the results of B-04 in patients with clinically negative nodes (Margolese, 1983). It is unlikely that less extensive surgery will improve overall survival. Therefore, other features involving psychological and social issues which influence the quality of life must be considered when evaluating the surgical approach.

Clinical trials for breast cancer surgery are particularly difficult to conduct. Individuality and the personal perception of surgical maneuvers in this field lead to a lack of uniformity in approach. In fact, in a recent survey of opinions from surgeons, principle investigators in NSABP trial B-06 which compares segmental mastectomy and postoperative radiation versus segmental mastectomy alone versus total mastectomy revealed the complexity of feelings involved (Taylor et al, 1984). These ranged from the concern of offending the doctor-patient relationship by participating in randomized clinical trials to the fear of personal responsibility if one treatment program turned out to be superior. Concerns about professional reputation and discussions involving uncertainty contribute to the reluctance of surgeons to participate in such a trial. Pre-consent randomization, in which treatment assignments are made prior to informing the patient and seeking consent (Zelen, 1980), was implemented in an attempt to increase patient entry in B-06 (Fisher et al, 1985a). Pre-consent randomization should only be used in special circumstances as an excess of patient or physician refusal to accept the assigned treatment will substantially reduce the impact of study findings.

Adjuvant treatment

Fortunately, the resistance regarding comparative studies of surgical procedures has not extended to investigations of adjuvant therapy for breast cancer. Most surgeons are willing to admit that surgery alone for breast cancer is not curative for all patients, and that additional therapy may be warranted for high risk patients. The decision regarding a recommendation of adjuvant therapy depends on the status of the *patient*, the extent and pathological characteristics of the *disease*, and the nature of the *treatments* which can be utilized. All three aspects of trials must be considered for the appropriate evaluation of therapy programs, and application of trial results to guide treatment decisions outside of trials.

The prognosis for patients with operable breast cancer is extremely variable. While possible prognostic factors have been suggested, clear cutoff points to objectively define risk groups have not been established. The variability of response to treatment and differences in tolerance and compliance also serve to make specific recommendations difficult. Thus, treatment programs and therapeutic objectives are often selected arbitrarily. Each physician weighs the risks and benefits of treatment according to a range of prognoses based on the patient and her disease. The worse the prognosis as ascertained by the surgeon, the greater the acceptable level of toxicity of adjuvant treatment. Patients in the more favorable prognostic subgroups may be considered unacceptable candidates for adjuvant therapy trials due to the high rate of surgical cure and the possiblitity to do harm with the added treatment. Establishing criteria to define suitable patient populations for treatment and study clarifies the objectives and acceptability of adjuvant therapy trials for breast cancer.

Studies of treatments for patients with advanced breast cancer provide an interesting contrast to those of adjuvant therapy. All patients have detectable manifestations of the disease so the rationale for some form of therapeutic intervention exists. Prognostic groups are easily distinguished based on the site of metastatic involvement. The objectives for treatment of patients with bone metastases alone (a protracted painful course) are undoubtedly different from those of patients with visceral involvement. The possibility for cure of patients with advanced disease is anecdotal. Thus, the intent of treatment for those patients must be considered palliative. The measurement of what can be defined as an effective therapy must be based on different criteria (many of them subjective) than the criteria used to evaluate adjuvant treatment. Issues of study design, sample size requirements, interpretation of results, and implications for the patient are also different.

The study of breast cancer, therefore, obliges the investigator to differentiate his view according to the detectable spread of the disease. Different questions and assessments will be dictated by the course of the disease. We discuss issues regarding protocol design, study conduct, treatment evaluation and drawing conclusions. *Our* conclusion is similar to Dr. Louis': the pursuit of truth requires great effort, care and diligence; it is not likely to be discovered by other means.

A clinical trial

We define a clinical trial as an *experiment* conducted with *human subjects* in which *treatments are initiated* for the purpose of *evaluating* one or more therapies. Our definition implies the existence of a prospective plan of action to be undertaken in the treatment of patients. We specifically exclude retrospective reviews as these do not involve the initiation of treatment for evaluation purposes.

A retrospective case review is not adequate to accurately characterize the impact of therapy. The choice of therapy and selection of the patient into the review may not be independent of the nature of the disease or of the outcome to be reported. If the last patient did well on a therapy, then the treatment may be repeated for the next patient. Otherwise, some other therapy would be attempted. When we look backward in time, we will not be able to reconstruct the treatment decision-making process and it will not be possible to describe the prescription for the future. In addition, if favorable results are obtained, it will not be possible to determine which factors may have influenced the outcome. There will be little uniformity and control of the aspects of the patients evaluated, the characterization of the disease or the treatments applied.

Requirement for study design

The *protocol document* describes a complete plan for the design and conduct of the clinical trial. The major components of the protocol are listed in Table 9.1. The list provides a guide to the main features which must be considered in clinical research.

The study schema summarizes all of the essential elements of the study design. It is a pictorial summary of the allocation of patients to the various treatments indicating the treatment programs and the timing of events.

A complete background section is required to ensure that all available results have been considered in the design of the study. Ethical principles dictate that patients not be placed at increased risk by participation in the study, and that there be a good chance for obtaining new and useful information. Without a thorough literature review, facts which form the basis for a sound study rationale may be overlooked.

Once the rationale for the study is firmly established, the specific objectives

Table 9.1 Outline of protocol document

Schema	— pictorial summary of the essentials of the study design. Should be simple and logical and reflect the study objectives.
Background	— prior results and rationale for the current study.
Objectives	— few in number, relate to schema, feasible.
Patient population	— clearly defined, ideally homogeneous.
Treatment allocation	— randomization to avoid bias, stratification to achieve balance, placebo control, crossover plan, etc.
Treatment	— give all details to describe administration, schedule, potential toxicities, dose modification, and duration. Use objective criteria to define the extent of surgical procedures.
Follow-up procedures	— schedules, clinical and laboratory data.
Endpoints	— standardize and quantify criteria for evaluating treatment effect.
Statistical considerations	— study design and sample size.
Forms submission	— simple, efficient, and comparable schedules for all treatment arms.
Informed consent	— risks, benefits, alternative treatments (including no additional therapy) and right to withdraw.

to be met by the current design need to be described. The objective should be stated as precisely as possible. Use of terms such as 'superior to' should be elaborated to describe the bases upon which superiority will be determined (e.g. improved relapse-free survival, reduction in toxic effects, better quality of life, etc.)

The patient population

Clear definition of the eligible patient population is a basic requirement for any well-conducted study. Patients who may be harmed by the treatment under study should not be entered; patients for whom standard effective therapies are available should also be excluded; and patients who are not likely to benefit from any of the treatments under study should not be included. Criteria for eligibility must be objective and identifiable at the time of study entry. At the conclusion of the trial, it must be clear to which patient population the study results might be extrapolated.

The definition of eligible patients must rely on conclusions drawn from existing data regarding the availability of 'effective' or 'ineffective' treatments. For example, sufficient data may be available to justify excluding patients with hormone receptor negative tumors from clinical trials which involve the evaluation of endocrine therapies. It is argued that including such patients in the trial may dilute our ability to detect treatment effects of the endocrine therapy by including a proportion of 'nonresponsive' patients in all treatment regimens. On the other hand, if the hormone receptor assay is not reliable, patients with true receptor positive tumors may be excluded, and the selection may change as the quality control of the laboratory changes. An alternative to excluding these patients would be to prospectively stratify the randomization and decide before conducting the trial that the results will be analyzed separately within patient subgroups defined by receptor status.

The variation in natural history of the disease for these patients is likely to be much larger than any observable differences in the effectiveness of treatment. Furthermore, the cutoff values for various features which may influence prognosis are not well established. Most of these factors influence prognosis along a continuum. For example, if a treatment is to be evaluated in high risk' patients, should those with four or more axillary lymph nodes involved be considered 'high risk'; or should ten or more positive nodes define 'high risk'? Ideally, we would like to establish a study sample of patients with as homogeneous an outcome as possible. However, by attempting to define a homogeneous population for which maximum benefit might be achieved with minimal risks, we might find that too few patients are available to enter the protocol sample to meet the required accrual objectives. There is a trade-off between narrowly defining eligible patients and achieving sample size objectives.

Treatments

The treatments to be applied in the study must be carefully defined so as to remove as much ambiguity as possible with respect to the prescription. Criteria for dose modification, and for delaying or stopping therapy should be established on objective bases. Doses, timing, schedule, and duration of medical treatment must be specified. Compliance testing procedures should also be considered. Potential risks and side effects should be stated and *corrective action* to be taken must also be given.

The acceptance of the prescribed treatment by the patient and the physician must be considered. This is particularly important in the adjuvant setting where treatment is administered to patients who do not have any signs or symptoms of the disease. Many of these patients may be unknowingly subjected to overtreatment. Thus, toxic effects and acceptance is an important issue for these apparently disease-free patients.

Prospective standardization of surgical procedures and pathological evaluations is also required. Terms such as radical mastectomy, modified radical mastectomy, axillary sampling, or axillary clearance should be avoided in the protocol document as different surgeons may associate different procedures with each of these terms. Instead, the extent of surgical procedures should be defined whenever possible using anatomical descriptors. For example, removal of the entire mammary gland and complete removal of all nodes in the axilla might define the extent of the minimal procedure required for patient entry into a particular adjuvant therapy protocol.

The role of randomization
Unfortunately, it is not possible to standardize and control all factors which might influence treatment outcome merely by careful definition in the protocol document. A fundamental principle in experimental sciences for comparing two treatments is that the groups must be alike in all aspects which are likely to affect outcome so that any observed differences might be attributable only to the treatment applied or to random variation. Any systematic bias making the groups noncomparable may lead to observed differences in treatment effect whereas no real differences exist. Similarly, real treatment differences may be missed if the comparison groups are not comparable. The term, *randomization*, refers to the use of a chance mechanism as a means for allocating treatments to patients. By giving each patient the same opportunity of receiving any of the therapies under investigation, the characteristics of the different treatment groups will be 'alike on the average' with respect to all factors which are likely to affect outcome. In this way, any observed differences in results between groups will tend to be due to the treatments.

Any comparative analyses for which the groups are established by mechanisms other than randomization may be subject to patient selection biases and/or environmental system biases. The former refer to differences in natural history prognosis, and characteristics of the disease or patients which are likely to influence the outcomes of treatment. These kinds of biases may be partially controlled by stratification of the analysis, matching techniques, and mathematical modeling, to compare treatment effects within more homogeneous subgroups of the patient population.

The environmental factor biases involve supportive care facilities, completeness of diagnostic work-up, aggressivity of treatment (philosophy of approach), training and experience of the surgeon, referral patterns, clinic waiting lists, quality and quantity of data collected, and any other feature characterizing the clinical setting of the investigation. These environmental biases cannot be corrected by sophisticated statistical modeling techniques and represent the major source of concern with respect to historically controlled analyses and analyses comparing treatment effects across studies. The biases due to environmental factors are largely nonquantifiable and therefore not amenable to corrective action. Only through prospective determination of control groups on the basis of some chance mechanism will these environmental factor biases be controlled 'on the average', making treatment comparisons unbiased within the trial.

We recognize that the use of randomization does not solve all of the difficulties in conducting clinical research on adjuvant therapies for breast cancer. Treatment groups may still be unbalanced with respect to prognostic factors within a single clinical trial. Furthermore, randomization helps to establish internal validity only, but does nothing to ensure that the protocol patients are representative of the larger population of interest. External validity, the appropriateness of extrapolating results from a clinical trial to the treatment of patients in standard clinical practice, is not established by randomization.

Several other techniques in addition to randomization are utilized to reduce the bias in comparisons of treatments. Often the randomization is stratified by factors which are felt to be prognostically important. Stratified randomization means that patients in different patient subpopulations are randomized separately so that an equal allocation of treatments to patients within a given strata can be guaranteed. Stratified randomization provides a control against the chance occurence of 'bad breaks' from the randomization, but in return adds an additional complexity to the treatment allocation process (Zelen, 1974; Peto et al, 1976).

Blinding is also used in the design of clinical trials to reduce biases of various types. Blinding refers to withholding information from the patient (single blind), patient and physician (double blind), or patient, physician and statistician (triple blind). The randomization is blinded so that physicians cannot select patients according to the treatment which will be allocated. Treatments are blinded so that any 'placebo effect' responses will be balanced across the regimens. Blinding of the evaluation process means that the individual determining the therapeutic response or examining the patient for possible recurrence is unaware of which treatment is being given. A recent study by the Eastern Cooperative Oncology Group (Cummings et al, 1984) compared tamoxifen versus placebo as adjuvant for patients 66 to 80 years old. Blinding of the reports on early study results allows study entry and progress to continue without being prejudiced by premature and possibly unreliable impressions. For reasons of safety, only a study monitoring committee need be aware of the early results.

Sample size considerations

The principal quantitative issues are described in the statistical considerations section of the protocol. The major study objectives in terms of the statistical endpoints to be measured are restated and preliminary plans for the statistical analysis of the data are presented. The required sample size is determined to guarantee the feasibility of the trial.

Four entities must be specified in order to determine the sample size requirements for a comparative clinical trial. First, the criteria for measuring treatment differences must be specified and the test statistic which will be used to compare treatment outcomes must be given. For example, the logrank procedure is commonly used for comparing treatment outcomes based on relapse-free survival, overall survival, or other measures evaluating time to an event of intetest. When recurrence or death (events) is the statistical endpoint of interest, statistical power is a function of the number of events observed rather than of the total number of patients entered.

The three remaining quantities (alpha, beta, delta) are shown in Table 9.2. For study design purposes, the table should be viewed within columns, i.e. vertically. Alpha is the acceptable false positive rate or type I error. This is the probability of deciding, based on the observed data (sample), that there is a treatment difference (for the entire population) when in fact no true treatment difference exists. Given that the correct answer is represented by the first column of the table, the mistake of deciding that there is a real treatment difference will be made only with the small probability of alpha. It has become standard practice to define alpha to be 0.05 or 0.01. These are two-sided if treatment differences in either direction would be considered worthy of reporting. For example, although a trial of adjuvant therapy versus a no-treatment control group would appear to represent a one-sided comparison (i.e. treatment is expected to improve outcome compared with no-treatment), it may be possible for the treatment to in fact have an adverse effect. Only if such an unexpected negative outcome from the treatment would never be interesting to report, is it reasonable to design the study as a one-sided comparison. Otherwise, sample sizes should be determined in order to provide adequate power to carry out two-sided tests of significance.

The quantities beta and delta are specified in the second column of the decision-truth table for the case when the treatment effects on the population

Table 9.2 The decision-truth table

		TRUTH	
		The Treatments Have Equal Efficacy (H_0 is True)	The Treatments Have Different Efficacy By An Amount $\triangle$ (H_0 is Not True)
DECISION	H_0 is True $(p > \alpha)$	O.K.	β-error Type II error
	H_0 is Not True $(p \leqslant \alpha)$	α-error Type I error	O.K. $1-\beta$ = Power

α is usually set at 0.05
For Design—View the table vertically
For Analysis—View the table horizontally

are really different. Delta is the magnitude of this difference between treatment outcomes. Beta is the probability that we will fail to decide that there is a difference based on our clinical trial. This beta error is referred to as a type II error. When the true treatment difference for the population is delta, the probability of deciding based on our clinical trial that there is a difference between the treatments is 1-beta. This is called the *statistical power* of the test to detect treatment differences as large as delta. As the delta of clinical significance gets small, the statistical power to detect this difference in the clinical trial decreases. For a fixed value of delta, the power can be increased by increasing the number of events within the sample. Therefore, given that a particular statistical endpoint and test procedure (logrank) will be used to evaluate treatment effects, the choices of alpha, beta and delta will determine the number of patients and events which are required to satisfy these criteria. For design purposes we set an accrual objective so that a clinically relevant difference (delta) will be detected with high probability (1–beta) when a decision rule designed to control alpha error (i.e. p. ≤ 0.05) is used.

Table 9.3 is reprinted from Freedman (1982) and shows the number of patients required using a logrank test to detect an improvement of delta = $P_2 - P_1$ in survival rate over a base line survival rate (P_1) for various two-sided alpha levels and statistical power requirements. The total number of patients and number of observed events required are given in this table. For example, 763 patients (343 deaths) are required in a trial designed to detect an improvement from 50–60% in survival rate with statistical power of 80% using a two-sided alpha = 0.05 logrank test. In studies of adjuvant therapy for breast cancer, treatment differences are likely to be, at best, in the 10–15% range, and overall survival rates are likely to be in the middle to upper ranges of the table. 300–700 + patients are required in order to adequately compare the effects of two treatments. In addition, patients who enter trials of adjuvant therapy for breast cancer must be followed for a long period of time in order to have a sufficient opportunity to observe enough events of interest.

Table 9.3 Number of patients (number of deaths) required to detect an improvement (P_2-P_1) in survival rate over a baseline survival rate (P_1) when: (i) alpha = 5%, 1-beta = 80%, (ii) alpha = 5%, 1-beta = 90%, (iii) alpha = 1%, 1-beta = 95%

			2-tailed logrank test		
			P_2-P_1		
P_1	0.05	0.10	0.15	0.20	0.35
	497 (459)	174 (156)	100 (87)	69 (59)	37 (28)
0.05	664 (615)	232 (209)	133 (116)	92 (78)	49 (38)
	1126 (1042)	393 (354)	225 (197)	156 (133)	82 (64)
	963 (843)	295 (251)	155 (128)	101 (80)	47 (34)
0.10	1289 (1128)	395 (335)	207 (171)	135 (108)	63 (45)
	2185 (1912)	668 (568)	351 (289)	228 (182)	105 (76)
	1415 (1167)	406 (325)	204 (158)	127 (95)	55 (37)
0.15	1894 (1562)	544 (435)	272 (211)	170 (128)	73 (49)
	3209 (2648)	921 (737)	461 (357)	288 (216)	123 (83)
	1827 (1416)	505 (379)	245 (178)	150 (105)	61 (38)
0.20	2445 (1895)	676 (507)	328 (238)	200 (140)	81 (51)
	4144 (3212)	1145 (858)	556 (403)	339 (237)	137 (85)

Table 9.3 (contd).

	2187 (1585)	589 (412)	280 (189)	168 (109)	65 (37)
0.25	2927 (2122)	788 (551)	375 (253)	224 (146)	87 (50)
	4961 (3597)	1335 (934)	634 (423)	380 (247)	147 (84)
	2487 (1679)	657 (427)	307 (192)	182 (109)	68 (36)
0.30	3330 (2247)	879 (571)	411 (257)	243 (145)	91 (47)
	5643 (3809)	1490 (968)	696 (435)	411 (246)	153 (80)
	2724 (1703)	709 (425)	327 (188)	191 (105)	70 (33)
0.35	3647 (2279)	949 (569)	438 (251)	255 (140)	93 (44)
	6181 (3863)	1607 (964)	741 (426)	432 (237)	156 (74)
	2895 (1665)	744 (409)	339 (178)	196 (98)	70 (29)
0.40	3876 (2228)	995 (547)	454 (238)	262 (131)	93 (39)
	6569 (3777)	1687 (927)	769 (403)	443 (221)	156 (66)
	2999 (1547)	762 (381)	344 (163)	197 (88)	68 (25)
0.45	4014 (2107)	1019 (509)	460 (218)	263 (118)	91 (34)
	6804 (3572)	1727 (863)	779 (370)	444 (200)	152 (57)
	3034 (1441)	763 (343)	341 (145)	193 (77)	65 (21)
0.50	4061 (1929)	1020 (459)	456 (193)	258 (103)	87 (28)
	6883 (3269)	1728 (777)	771 (327)	436 (174)	145 (47)
	3001 (1275)	746 (298)	330 (123)	185 (64)	61 (17)
0.55	4017 (1707)	998 (399)	441 (165)	247 (86)	81 (22)
	6808 (2893)	1691 (676)	746 (280)	417 (146)	135 (37)
	2900 (1087)	713 (249)	312 (101)	173 (52)	56 (12)
0.60	3881 (1455)	953 (333)	417 (135)	231 (69)	74 (16)
	6577 (2466)	1615 (565)	705 (229)	389 (116)	122 (27)
	2730 (887)	663 (198)	286 (78)	157 (39)	
0.65	3654 (1187)	886 (265)	382 (105)	209 (52)	
	6192 (2012)	1500 (450)	646 (177)	352 (88)	
	2493 (685)	596 (149)	253 (57)	137 (27)	
0.70	3337 (917)	796 (199)	338 (76)	182 (36)	
	5654 (1555)	1347 (336)	570 (128)	306 (61)	
	2190 (492)	512 (102)	214 (37)	114 (17)	
0.75	2930 (659)	684 (136)	284 (49)	150 (22)	
	4965 (1117)	1157 (231)	478 (83)	250 (37)	
	1821 (318)	413 (62)	168 (21)		
0.80	2436 (426)	551 (82)	222 (27)		
	4125 (722)	930 (139)	371 (46)		
	1387 (173)	300 (30)			
0.85	1854 (231)	398 (39)			
	3138 (392)	668 (66)			
	892 (66)				
0.90	1189 (89)				
	2007 (150)				

Reproduced with permission from Freedman (1982).

Requirement for cooperative trials

Because of the large number of patients required to carry out these studies, it is extremely rare to find a sufficient number available for study within a single institution. Comparative evaluations of therapies for adjuvant breast cancer can, therefore, only be carried out in multi-center trials. New approaches can and should be developed, fine-tuned, and piloted within single institutions. However, the results should not be extrapolated as a recommendation for treatment of a larger population until an adequately controlled, statistically powerful clinical trial is conducted. The natural history of breast cancer is so variable and the factors other than treatment which are likely to influence outcome so great, that the results accumulated from the treatment of a series of patients are not likely to be precisely reproducible from occasion to occasion. Using randomization to establish comparison groups will reduce the possibility for claiming major therapeutic impact which is overly optimistic.

Conducting the trial

Attention to detail and concern for the control of bias also apply to the execution of the study. Protocol treatments must be delivered according to prescription provided this continues to be in the interest of the patient. Regular follow-up visits are required to maintain uniformity in control of treatment compliance and standardization regarding the times at which recurrences might be detected. Asymptomatic relapses may be detected as first recurrence site for patients who are followed regularly, while painful recurrences might appear to be more common for patients who are not on a regular follow-up schedule. The thoroughness of follow-up evaluation and the reporting of findings must be comparable for all treatment programs being evaluated.

Clinical endpoints are patient conditions which dictate a change in treatment program, i.e. at relapse. These should be distinguished from statistical endpoints which are criteria to be used for evaluating the impact of therapy. Some confusion exists regarding the meaning of the phrase 'off protocol'. From a clinical point of view, this phrase means that the patient is no longer being cared for under the protocol specified treatment regimen assigned. However, it does not mean that the patient is no longer to be followed, as the statistical endpoint of evaluation of overall survival requires that all patients be followed as study patients until the time of death. Thus, 'off protocol treatment' does not mean 'off protocol study'.

The type, format and quality of data collected should match the study objectives and purposes of the analysis. Data specifically for the main treatment comparisons should be collected in a uniform format with supporting documentation provided as background. Self-coding, computer compatible forms reduce transcription errors and speed data processing. Baseline data on the patient and her disease, on the treatments actually received, toxic effects, and outcome measures are required.

Data quality control procedures should be established to ensure that coded results are consistent, complete, and accurate. Centralized data, pathology and laboratory reviews are requirements for trials of adjuvant therapy for breast cancer.

Therapy evaluation

Objective criteria need to be established as a measure of the impact of therapy. In studies involving patients with operable breast cancer, overall survival (OS) has been adopted as the ultimate criteria by which therapies are evaluated. Long follow-up periods are required in order to obtain good estimates of OS. Relapse-free survival (RFS) measures the time from operation to the recurrence of breast cancer. RFS has been assumed to be an early indicator of ultimate survival experience so that treatments providing improved RFS were considered to benefit the patient. Unfortunately, prolonged RFS has not resulted in improved OS within most of the adjuvant therapy trials reported to date. Substantially longer follow-up might be required before any difference in OS might be observed.

RFS provides an overly optimistic evaluation of the impact of therapy by considering patients who die without definitive evidence of breast cancer and those who develop a second malignancy as non-failures in the analysis (Kay & Schumacher, 1983). Some deaths without recurrence might be due to the treatment itself, and others might be found with disease if autopsy had been performed. In order to reduce the overly optimistic evaluation of treatment effect, we recommend that disease-free survival (DFS) be reported in which patients who die are counted as failures (Ludwig Group, 1984).

A common error is made by reporting the distribution of site of first relapse considering as the denominator only patients who failed. The information gained from such an analysis is conditional on knowing prospectively which patients will relapse. A meaningful evaluation which reflects the impact of therapy upon patterns of relapse for the entire population should be made using the entire study sample as the denominator.

Not all sites of relapse have the same subsequent prognosis. While patients who have systemic failure are known to have a predictable dire prognosis, those with isolated mastectomy scar recurrence alone or those with operable cancer in the contralateral breast will have a less predictable outcome. Therefore, evaluation of systemic disease-free survival (SDFS) may provide a better indicator for ultimate overall survival than RFS (Ludwig Group, 1984).

Case exclusions

When a clinical trial has been conducted and the data are ready to analyze, investigators may wish to exclude from the analysis some of the patients who were entered on the study. Two points of view can be applied to determine case exclusion (Sackett & Gent, 1979). With the *explanatory* point of view, only patients who meet precise criteria for evaluability and who receive the treatment programs precisely as defined in the protocol are included in the analysis. The intent is to define the effects of treatment under ideal circumstances for the main purposes of generating hypotheses and establishing criteria for future study. In contrast, the *management or pragmatic* approach is that all patients who enter a clinical trial should be included in the analysis according to the principle of 'intent to treat'. The evaluation of the treatment policy is the main purpose of such an analysis.

Case exclusion on the basis of factors which might be treatment or disease dependent may cause the group of patients remaining for analysis to be non-representative and the results to be biased with respect to application of the therapies to the entire population. For example, patients assigned to receive adjuvant chemotherapy but who fail to receive full doses may be excluded from an analysis. The exclusion criteria will not apply to patients assigned to receive no adjuvant therapy. If the excluded patients tend to have a worse prognosis, then the patients in the evaluated chemotherapy group will have a better crude prognosis than those in the no adjuvant treatment group. Adjuvant chemotherapy will appear to be better when, in fact, the effect is due to differences in prognosis for the patients who are left for the analysis. The protection against bias provided by the randomization will thus be lost.

'Statistical proof': What does it mean?

Many investigators take the results of clinical trials as representing a proof of a hypothesis of interest. Table 9.2 when considered horizontally represents the decision-making criteria applied at the time of analysis. The standard way of evaluating statistical evidence is to compute a p-value which indicates the probability of obtaining the observed treatment differences (plus differences more extreme than those observed), if we pretend that the treatments really have equivalent effects when given to the total population. The usual convention is to consider $p \leq 0.05$ as an indication that the treatments may not produce equivalent effects. The rationale for this interpretation is that p-values ≤ 0.05 occur only rarely by chance alone. If $p \leq 0.05$, then we decide that the treatments are different as indicated by the bottom row in Table 9.2. It is possible that the treatments have identical therapeutic effects (the first column of Table 9.2), and that we, in fact, observed a rare event. Thus, obtaining $p \leq 0.05$ does not prove that the treatments have different effects. Similarly, if we obtain $p > 0.05$ (top row of Table 9.2), it is possible that the treatments really have effects which differ by an amount delta (second column of Table 9.2), but that our trial failed to detect this difference due to a high beta error. Thus, failure to demonstrate a statistically significant difference also does not prove that the treatments really have equivalent effects. Therefore, conducting a well-designed clinical trial can only provide convincing evidence for or against treatment differences.

Interpretation and conclusions from analyses of subgroups
A common practice is to devote a large part of a report on clinical trials to the analysis of treatment effects within various subgroups of the patients in the study. Such analyses of treatment effects within multiple subgroups have an increased likelihood of finding a false positive effect by virtue of the multiplicity of analyses. If the data analysis within each subgroup has a 5% possibility to achieve statistical significance by chance alone, the chance of finding *at least one* significant result within some subgroup is much greater than the nominal value of 5%. In addition, multiple subgroup analyses increase the chance that a spurious treatment-subgroup interaction effect might be indicated. Therefore, when such effects are found in the data, we should report the findings, but not believe them (Peto, 1983).

The investigator's desire to evaluate treatment effects within subgroups of the patient population is a manifestation of his desire to treat the individual patient with the best available regimen designed specifically for the individual. This desire is in conflict with the main research capabilities of the clinical trial. Unfortunately, analysis of patient subgroups within a clinical trial have a high risk of producing false positive results. Furthermore, subdividing the patient population will result in two few patients remaining for analysis in any specific subgroup. Finally, if the results of subgroup analyses are taken incorrectly as 'statistical proof' of a treatment effect, physicians may find it difficult to withhold apparently effective treatment, and the reconfirmation of the initial findings may become impossible. Subgroup analyses of clinical trials data should be performed to generate research hypotheses and to gain insights regarding the possible mechanism of actions of therapies. However, such analyses should not be used to tailor-make treatment for the individual patient without reconfirmation of findings from additional sources. The results from the overall study population should remain the major component of the report on a treatment advance.

Quality of life

Measurement of quality of life may be one of the most important considerations to infer the impact of therapy for the individual patient. The quality of one's life is a philosophical issue depending on the angle of view, the treatment, the disease and the environment in which the patient lives and in which the measurement is made. Performance status as assessed by the doctor in advanced disease applications restricts the patient's viewpoint and provides a somewhat objective measure of life quality. This assessment of functional status has been verified as a prognostic factor (Yates et al, 1980).

Other methods of measurement, such as the appearance of the patient to the physician or an expression by the patient regarding her own sense of well-being, are not readily reproducible and provide little standardization to enable extrapolation of the value of the measurement to other patients. The linear analogue self-assessment (LASA) is the most commonly used method for assessing some aspects concerning the quality of life for cancer patients (Coates et al, 1983). This technique is the basis for a Functional Living Index—Cancer (Schipper et al, 1984) recently developed and validated. The prognostic utility of this index has yet to be determined. A simple statement from the patient (poor, moderate, good) about her perceived life quality may be sufficient to assess the impact of the therapy. As in melanoma (Rogentine et al, 1979), we may find that patients with breast cancer who claim they cope well with the disease are living longer. The psychological and social aspects involved with the diagnosis and treatment of breast cancer are far from being completely focused. The anxiety related to the diagnosis, the psychological morbidity of mastectomy, the role of adjuvant therapy and follow-up in reminding the patient of her disease are only some of the issues currently being investigated (Maguire et al, 1983).

The requirement for clinical trials

Assessment of the currently available treatment approaches for breast cancer is not possible by retrospective review of cases. The magnitude of the therapeutic advances which can be anticipated are so small, and the patient population so heterogenous that a retrospective comparison between two groups of women with breast cancer is destined to be inaccurate (Baum & Berstock, 1982). Large numbers of patients followed for long periods of time are required to identify moderate but clinically relevant advances in therapeutic outcome. Standardization of the patient population, treatment programs, data collection procedures, and evaluation of endpoints is required to remove biases which can influence the statistical inferences. The use of randomization as a means for assigning treatments to patients establishes comparison groups which are 'alike on the average', and helps control for both conscious and unconscious biases. Quality control of treatment, compliance, follow-up schedules and centralized review of data are essential to describe the actual conduct of the trial. Only by careful attention to the rigorous requirements of scientific investigation, can we avoid establishing inadequate therapies as standards for the treatment of patients with breast cancer.

REFERENCES

Baum M, Berstock D 1982 Breast cancer—adjuvant therapy. Clinics in Oncology 1: 901–915
Berkeley G 1752 Farther thoughts on tar-water. In: Fraser A C (ed) 1901 The works of George Berkeley, Vol. 3, Clarendon Press, Oxford
Bonchek L I 1979 Are randomized trials appropriate for evaluating new operations? New England Journal of Medicine 301: 44–45
Bull J P 1959 The historical development of clinical therapeutic trials. Journal of Chromic Diseases 10: 215–248
Coates A, Fischer Dillenbeck C, McNeil D R, et al 1983 On the receiving end-II. Linear analogue self-assessment (LASA) in evaluation of aspects of the quality of life of cancer patients receiving therapy. European Journal of Cancer Clinical Oncology 19: 1633–1637
Cummings F, Gray R, Davis T et al 1984 Double blind adjuvant therapy with tamoxifen versus placebo in patients older than 65 years with Stage II breast cancer. Proccedings ASCO Abstract C-490, Toronto
Fisher B, Bauer M, Margolese R, et al 1985a Five-year results of a randomized clinical trial comparing total mastectomy and segmental mastectomy with or without radiation in the treatment of breast cancer. New England Journal of Medicine 312: 665–673
Fisher B, Redmond C, Fisher E R, et al 1985b Ten-year results of a randomized clinical trial comparing radical mastectomy and total mastectomy with or without radiation. New England Journal of Medicine 312: 674–681
Freedman L S 1982 Tables of the number of patients required in clinical trials using the logrank test. Statistics in Medicine 1: 121–129
Kaplan E L, Meier P 1958 Nonparametric estimation from incomplete observations. Journal of the American Statistical Association 53: 457–481
Kay R, Schumacher M 1983 Unbiased assessment of treatment effects on disease recurrence and survival in clinical trials. Statistics in Medicine 2: 41–59
Lectures on Statistical Science for Oncologists, Division of Biostatistics and Epidemiology, Dana-Farber Cancer Institute, Boston 1979
Lind J 1753 A treatise of the scurvy. Sands Murray and Cochran, Edinburgh
Lister J 1870 On the effects of the antiseptic system upon the salubrity of a surgical hospital. Lancet i, 4 and 40
Louis P C A 1834 Essay on clinical instruction (trans.) Martin P, London
Louis P C A 1836 Researches on the effects of blood-letting (trans.), Putnam C G, Boston

Ludwig Breast Cancer Study Group 1984 Randomized trial of chemo-endocrine therapy, endocrine therapy and mastectomy alone in postmenopausal patients with operable breast cancer and axillary node metastasis. Lancet i: 1256–1260

Maguire P, Van Dam F 1983 Psychological aspects of breast cancer; workshop report. European Journal of Cancer Clinical Oncology 19: 1735–1740

Margolese R G 1983 Choice for primary surgery. In: Margolese R G (ed) Breast cancer. Churchill Livingstone, New York p 77–92

Mike V 1982 Clinical studies in cancer: a historical perspective. In: Mike V, Stanley K E (eds) Statistics in Medical Research, John Wiley and Sons, New York, p. 111–155

National Surgical Adjuvant Breast Project 1983 Report on Protocol B-06, Group Minutes.

Peto R 1982 Chapter 44. In: Halnan K (ed) Treatment of Cancer, Chapman and Hall, London, p 867–871

Peto R, Pike M C, Armitage P, et al 1976 Design and analysis of randomized clinical trials requiring prolonged observation of each patient: I. Introduction and design. British Journal of Cancer 34: 585–612

Peto R, Pike M C, Armitage P, et al 1977 Design and analysis of randomized clinical trials requiring prolonged observation of each patient: II. Analysis and examples. British Journal of Cancer 35: 1–39

Pocock S J 1983 Clinical trials: A practical approach. John Wiley and Sons, Chichester

Rogentine G N, van Kammen D P, Fox B H et al 1979 Psychological factors in the prognosis of malignant melanoma: a prospective study. Psychosomatic Medicine 4(8): 647–655

Sackett D, Gent M 1979 Controversy in counting and attributing events in clinical trials. New England Journal of Medicine 301: 1410–1412

Schipper H, Clinch J, McMurray A, Levitt M 1984 Measuring the quality of life of cancer patients: The functional living index—cancer: Development and validation. Journal of Clinical Oncology 2: 472–483

Taylor K M, Margolese R G, Soskolne C L 1984 Physicians' reasons for not entering patients in a randomized clinical trial of surgery for breast cancer. New England Journal of Medicine 310: 1363–1367

Veronesi U, Saccozzi R, DelVecchio M et al 1981 Comparing radical mastectomy with quadrantectomy, axillary dissection, and radiotherapy in patients with small cancers of the breast. New England Journal of Medicine 305: 6–11

Yates J W, Chalmer B, McKegney F P 1980 Evaluation of patients with advanced cancer using the Karnofsky Performance Status. Cancer 45: 2220–2224

Zelen M 1974 The randomization and stratification of patients to clinical trials. Journal of Chronic Diseases 27: 365–375

Zelen M 1982 Strategy and alternate randomized designs in cancer clinical trials. Cancer Treatment Reports 66: 1095–1100

Zelen M 1983 Guidelines for publishing papers on cancer clinical trials: Responsibilities of editors and authors. Journal of Clinical Oncology 1: 164–169

10 Adjuvant chemotherapy trials in breast cancer: an appraisal and lessons for patient care outside the trials

ARON GOLDHIRSCH, RICHARD
D. GELBER AND BEN W. DAVIS

Introduction

Since this paper was written, updates have appeared for some cited studies, and some other results have been newly reported. An overview of data on mortality by allocated treatment has been performed based on more than 16 000 women randomized into trials with tamoxifen and more than 10 000 women randomized into chemotherapy trials. The analysis indicated that among women with early breast cancer there was a statistically significant reduction in short-term mortality for those receiving either form of adjuvant therapy (BCTG/UICC/WHO, 1984). The precise magnitude of the benefit in terms of time gained and the clinical significance of these results have yet to be determined. These data do not alter the conclusions of this report.

Adjuvant drug treatment (chemotherapy and/or endocrine therapy) has become commonplace in the management of breast cancer despite the fact that its merit has yet to be definitely established (NIH consensus statement, 1980). Randomized clinical trials concerning operable breast cancer have provided answers to certain of the outstanding questions. Were an overall judgment to be made of the present status of adjuvant therapy, and guidelines to emerge on the basis of such judgment, it would have to be concluded that no significant breakthrough in curative treatment has been achieved. Further clinical trials must pursue more effective treatments and a more comprehensive understanding of breast cancer.

In the absence of standard definitions of patient populations (eligible, evaluable, etc.) and endpoints (disease-free survival, relapse-free survival, etc.), a review of the treatment results of adjuvant therapy trials must take into account a broad spectrum of logical assumptions and extrapolated conclusions. Moreover, clinical trials in breast cancer require large numbers of patients followed for long periods of time in order to provide meaningful results and conclusions. The natural history of operable breast cancer is such that 10% of operated patients will die each year (Baum, 1982a; Hellman, 1982). Over 100 deaths must be observed in order for there to be a good chance of statistical detection of a decrease in mortality as great as 50% after treatment. However, the experience of recent years seems to limit the probable overall survival

123

advantage with available treatments to 10–20% over that of untreated populations (Baum, 1982b). Thus, larger trials are required for discernment of such advances. In considering lessons to be learned from clinical trials in adjuvant breast cancer, it would have been beneficial to present the data in terms of recommendations for patient subpopulations. The physician's index for selecting appropriate treatment is based on the characteristics of the host and the disease being treated. With this information the choice of treatment is then made. Unfortunately, the details required to make such a presentation are not readily available from the literature. The research perspective is oriented toward comparison of treatment programs rather than toward recommendations for defined patient subpopulations. In addition, analyses of treatment results within subgroups are hazardous, as they are likely to produce significant findings by chance alone. A cautious approach to the interpretation of subgroup analyses needs to be adopted, as suggested by others (Peto 1982): '. . . If we find one subgroup in which most of the treatment benefit appears to be concentrated, and such a subgroup can almost always be found, then note and report this fact but do not believe it. . . .'.

The best way to confirm the validity of such an observation is by comparative analysis of the data from other similar trials to determine if the findings are repeated. As more evidence accumulates and analyses based on prior hypotheses are confirmatory, the unexpected finding may be established as representative of a real treatment effect. A further problem in defining appropriate treatments for individual patients from results of clinical trials is that patients who enter trials are preselected for inclusion and might not be representative of the total population having the disease. If a trial is a randomized comparative study, the results will be internally valid in that outcome differences will reflect real treatment effects on the average for the type of patient entered into the trial. The external validity for extrapolating the effect of treatment on future patients may be questionable if the study patients are not representative.

Nevertheless, an evaluation of the results available from randomized prospective controlled trials may generate conclusions which can be applied to the treatment of patients with breast cancer. It should be stressed that since *no* breakthrough has been achieved to date in the treatment of operable breast cancer, efforts must be made to enter patients into controlled, well designed and well documented trials, in the interests of determining more effective therapy for future patients.

Trials with a mastectomy-alone (or placebo) control group

The results of seven trials with a mastectomy-alone control arm and adjuvant treatment with chemotherapy have been reported. In two of these trials, one by the NSABP (Fisher et al, 1980) and the other at Guy's Hospital (Rubens et al, 1983), adjuvant treatment was by oral melphalan for the duration of two years. In four trials a combination chemotherapy with an alkylating agent (cyclophosphamide or chlorambucil) together with anti-metabolites (methotrexate and 5-fluorouracil) was used. These four trials show a significant advantage in favor of the adjuvant treatment in terms of relapse-free survival (RFS) at the reported follow-up time. In a trial carried out in Manchester the combination with cyclophosphamide, methotrexate and 5-fluoro-uracil (CMF) was compared with single-agent chemotherapy with melphalan (L-PAM) and with a mastectomy-alone control group. Significant advantages in terms of RFS for the CMF as compared to the other two groups were observed. The use of a five-drug combination in which adriamycin and vincris-tine were added to a CMF regimen yielded similar results. No advantage in terms of overall survival (OS) has been reported in any of these trials (Table 10.1).

It would be necessary to compare the results of these trials in order to learn the lesson concerning the role of chemotherapy in operable breast cancer with axillary lymph node metastases. Unfortunately, this cross-study analysis cannot be done without the possibility of distorted conclusions, since the patient popu-lations are not uniform in initial prognosis, there is often institutional varia-bility in selection of patients, and the methods used in reporting results are not standard. Nevertheless, a consistent finding is that systemic therapy with cytotoxic drugs produces a benefit in disease-free survival and a modest (10–20%) benefit in overall survival for premenopausal patients with a low tumor burden (small primary and low number of axillary lymph nodes involved). Detection of these modest differences in treatment results at an acceptable level of statistical power requires the accrual of large numbers of patients (Boag et al, 1971). The 2203 evaluated patients in these seven trials received five different types of chemotherapy regimens or surgery alone, distributed among eight treatment groups and seven control groups. On the whole the trials have consistently shown a real, though limited, benefit from treatment with cytotoxic drugs for the overall population of studied patients with operable breast cancer and axillary metastases.

Trials with a melphalan-treated control group

Nine trials produced data for comparisons of a combination of an alkylating agent (cyclophosphamide or melphalan) and one or more anti-metabolites (5-fluorouracil and/or methotrexate) with melphalan. In two trials vincristine and/or prednisone were added to the chemotherapy combination. Most of the 2215 patients evaluated in these nine trials had lymph node metastases (Table 10.2). All but one of the trials (University of Alabama) showed an advantage in terms of RFS for treatment with a combination of drugs. The results of the SWOG trial, which compared an aggressive five-drug combination with a single drug, showed a RFS and an OS advantage for the patients treated with the combination.

The trials using melphalan as a control treatment have generally shown a statistically significant difference in outcome favoring the more aggressive (and usually more toxic) treatments. In five of the trials the subpopulation of post-menopausal women derived the most benefit from the combination.

Table 10.1 Trials with a mastectomy-alone control group

Trial, (Reference) population	Investigated treatments	Reported follow-up	OVERALL relevant findings		Largest most benefitting subpopulation
			DFS/RFS	OS	
NSABP (Fisher et al, 1975b, 1984) pre & post; N+	L-PAM	10 years	N.S.	N.S.	$\leq$49 years old: significant benefit in RFS + OS (p = 0.02 and 0.05 respectively)
GUYS (Rubens et al, 1983) pre & post; N+	L-PAM	5 years	N.S.	N.S.	1–3 N+: advantage not statistically significant (p = 0.08)
Manchester (Howat et al, 1981) pre & post; N+, T_{3A} N_0	L-PAM CMF	3 years	N.S. p = 0.0004	— —	postmenopausal: significant benefit for CMF over L-PAM and controls
Milano (Bonadonna et al, 1984) pre & post; N+	CMF	9 years	p < 0.001	N.S.	premenopausal: significant benefit in RFS & OS (p = 0.0005 and 0.02 respectively)
OSAKO (Senn et al, 1984) pre & post; N+	LMF(+BCG)	7 years	p = 0.01	N.S.	postmenopausal: significant benefit in RFS but not in OS
MBCCG (Wheeler, 1979) pre & post clin. N_{1A+B}	CMF/(VM)	3 years	p = 0.01	—	—
West Midlands (Morrison et al, 1984) pre & post; N+	AVCMF (+leucovorin)	3 3/4 years	p = 0.04	N.S.	premenopausal patients: significant benefit in RFS (p = 0.02)

pre: premenopausal
post: postmenopausal
L-PAM: Melphalan

C: cyclophosphamide
M: methotrexate
F: 5-fluorouracil

L: chlorambucil
V: Vincristine
A: Adriamycin

DFS/RFS: Disease or relapse free survival
OS: Overall survival
N.S.: Not significant

Table 10.2 Trials with a melphalan (L-PAM) treated control group

Trial, (Reference) population	Investigated Treatments	Reported follow-up	OVERALL relevant findings		Largest most benefitting subpopulation
			DFS/RFS	OS	
NSABP (Fisher et al, 1980) pre & post; N+	L-PAM + F	4 years	N.S.	N.S.	≥50 years old and N+ 4: significant benefit in RFS & OS
SWOG (Rivkin et al, 1984a) Pre & post; N+,	CMFVP	5 years	p = 0.002	p = 0.002	All N+ 1–3: reported significant advantage in RFS and OS
Manchester (Howat et al, 1981) Pre & post; N+, T_3N_0	CMF	3 years	p = 0.03	N.S.	postmenopausal: significant benefit in RFS
COG (Davis et al, 1979) Pre & post; N+ (some N−)	CMF-V	4 years	p = 0.003	N.S.	postmenopausal ≥50 years old benefit in RFS
Univ. of Alabama (Carpenter et al, 1982) Pre & post; N+	CMF	3 years	N.S.	p = 0.026	(in favour of L-PAM treatment!!)
Bowman Gray (Cooper et al, 1981) Pre & post; N+	CMF (±RT)	2 years	p = 0.05	N.S.	≥50 years old: significant benefit in RFS
Northwest Univ. (Caprini et al, 1980) Pre & post; N+	CFP (±RT)	2 years	p = 0.01	N.S.	postmenopausal: significant benefit in RFS
Mayo (Ahman et al, 1978) Pre & post; N+, Txb of T_4	CFP (±RT)	2 years	p = 0.01	N.S.	premenopausal: significant benefit in RFS
Fox Chase (Creech et al, 1983) Pre & post; N+	CMF	ongoing(?)	N.S.	N.S.	premenopausal: borderline benefit in RFS (p = 0.056)

Table 10.3 Trials with a CMF treated control group

Trial, (Reference) population	Investigated Treatments	Reported follow-up	OVERALL relevant findings		Largest most benefitting subpopulation
			DFS/RFS	OS	
CALGB (Tormey et al, 1983) pre & post; N+	CMFVP CMF + MER	4 years	$p < 0.01$ N.S.	N.S. N.S.	postmenopausal: significant benefit in RFS —
ECOG (Tormey et al, 1984) Premenopausal N+	CMFP* + T CMFP	3 years	N.S. N.S.	— —	N+ $\geq$4: DFS ($p = 0.09$) None
LBCS I premenop.; N+ (n°1–3 N+)	CMFp**	3 years	N.S.	N.S.	None

* P = 'high-dose' prednisone (40 mg/m^2 daily on days 1–14 each cycle)
** p = 'low-dose' prednisone (7.5 mg daily continuously)

Trials with a CMF-combination-treated control group

The observation that the CMF combination was superior to melphalan led to the development of trials using this treatment in the control group (Table 10.3). 1499 patients have been evaluated in the trials using CMF as a control for comparisons. The following three observations have been made:

(1) The more aggressive and more toxic CMFVP combination therapy was associated with a RFS benefit (but not an OS advantage); this was due to a longer RFS in the postmenopausal subpopulation (p=0.02) but not in the premenopausal patients (p=0.09).

(2) Premenopausal patients do not seem to gain any survival benefit from the addition of low- or high-dose prednisone, although the average CMF dose administered has been significantly higher if given with prednisone.

(3) At 3 years of median follow-up the results of treatment with the addition of tamoxifen to the adjuvant chemotherapy of premenopausal patients were similar to those attained with CMF or CMFP.

Trials with combined endocrine and chemotherapy

The combination of endocrine therapy and chemotherapy had its origin in the hypothesis that treatment results would be improved if the two modalities were used simultaneously. Results in the adjuvant setting are available from seven studies (Table 10.4). Five trials were created to evaluate the combination of the two modalities as compared with a chemotherapy alone; two of these used oophorectomy and chemotherapy as the combined modality treatment. In two further trials the combination of endocrine and chemotherapy was compared to endocrine therapy alone (LBCS III and SWOG), while a mastectomy-alone control group is included in only one trial (LBCS III). The preliminary conclusions from this heterogeneous set of trials must be considered separately. Two factors have emerged as indicators of endocrine treatment outcome, i.e. menopausal status and steroid hormone receptor content of the primary tumor.

In postmenopausal patients the addition of tamoxifen to an adjuvant combination chemotherapy might be adequate for patients with unknown tumor hormone receptor content. In patients with tumors containing high estrogen or progesterone receptor content, it is unclear whether combination chemotherapy adds to the benefit obtained from endocrine therapy alone. In postmenopausal patients with PR-negative tumors a detrimental effect resulting from the addition of tamoxifen to chemotherapy has been suggested by one investigator (Fisher et al, 1984), but as yet not confirmed by another (Tormey et al, 1984).

Premenopausal patients younger than 50 years did not benefit from the addition of tamoxifen (T) to melphalan and 5-fluorouracil (PF). At a median

Table 10.4 Randomized Trials with a combination endocrine and chemotherapy

Trial (Reference) population	Investigated Treatments	Reported follow-up	OVERALL relevant findings DFS	OS	Largest most benefitting subpopulation
NSABP (Fisher et al, 1983b) Pre & post N+	L-PAM + F L-PAM + F + T	3 years		N.S.	≥50 years old: significant benefit in RFS; N+ 4 also OS NEGATIVE EFFECT in OS in prem. with Progesterone receptor negative tumors
ECOG (Tormey et al, 1984) Pre N+	CMFP CMFP + T	3 years	N.S.	—	N+ ≥4: trends in favour of the T combination
ECOG (Tormey et al, 1984) Post N+	observation CMFP CMFP + T	3 years	N.S.	—	ER-: RFS benefit for CMFP/CMFP+T vs obs
Case Western (Hubay et al, 1981) Pre & Post N+	CMF CMFT (± BCG)	4 years	N.S.	—	Patients with ER+: significant benefit in RFS
LBCS III (Ludwig Group, 1984) Post N+	p + T vs obs CMFp + T vs obs	3 years	p = 0.008 p < 0.001	N.S.	Trial dealing with young (age≤65 years) post ER+: no benefit of CMFp+T over p + T (DFS) ER-: no difference between p + T and obs (DFS)
LBCS II Pre N+ 4	CMFp Ox + CMFp	3 years	N.S.	N.S.	none
SWOG (Rivkin et al, 1984b) Post N+, ER+	CMFVP T CMFVp + T	3 years (ongoing)	N.S.	—	none
SWOG (Rivkin et al, 1984b) Pre N+, ER+	CMFVP Ox + CMFVP	3 years (ongoing)	p = 0.055	—	none

obs: observation surgery alone control
Ox: Oophorectomy

of 36 months an overall survival disadvantage (64% for PFT vs 87% for PF; p=0.001) indicated that tamoxifen might be detrimental for patients *without* steroid hormone receptors in the primary tumors. Although a survival disadvantage was also seen for patients in the same age group with ER-negative tumors, regardless of the PR status, the presence of PR was shown to be more predictive of treatment outcome. Patients with ER-positive but PR-negative tumors had a DFS (p=0.03) and a survival disadvantage (p=0.01) when tamoxifen was added to the PF combination. Another similar trial (ECOG) did not show the same results: no difference at a median follow-up time of three years was noted between premenopausal patients who had received chemotherapy alone and those who had received chemotherapy plus tamoxifen.

Two trials, one of them in progress (LBCS II and the ongoing SWOG trial for ER+ premenopausal patients), are designed to test the effectiveness of oophorectomy added to a combination chemotherapy. While minimal differences in DFS between treatment groups in the SWOG trial have been noted, it is too early to draw conclusions from the preliminary results. In contrast, LBCS II was designed to test the addition of oophorectomy in a high-risk premenopausal population (≥ 4 N+). In this setting, no difference between treatment groups has been detected at four years of median follow-up.

Until new data emerge from evaluation of ongoing or terminated trials the role of adjuvant combined chemo- and endocrine therapy will remain controversial.

The duration of treatment

Results are available from five trials in which the main question concerned duration of treatment initiated after healing of the mastectomy wound (Table 10.5). The shortest therapy investigated thus far is one lasting 15 weeks, and no differences in outcome were shown between this duration and a treatment of 30 weeks. The results of these trials (Table 10.5) suggest that shortening the duration of the therapies tested to six months (or 4 months as in the DFCI trial) does not alter the outcome obtainable from a longer duration of administration of the same drugs. Whether this applies to all subgroups remains unknown.

The question of timing of drug administration

A variety of experiments, involving both drug administration in animal models of breast cancer (Fisher et al, 1983a) and mathematical models of solid tumor growth (Goldie J H, 1980) have provided a biological rationale for early administration of adjuvant chemotherapy. The 15-year results of the Scandinavian Adjuvant Chemotherapy Study Group (SACSG) strongly suggest that the effectiveness of adjuvant chemotherapy may be enhanced by administration in the perioperative period (Nissen-Meyer et al, 1978). These results must be confirmed as the treatment groups in this study may not be well-balanced for prognostic factors. Answers may emerge from the other controlled trials (Table 10.6). Two retrospectively analyzed non-randomized trials deserve comment. Cooper et al (1979) reported that the efficacy of the five-drug regimen, CMFVP (cyclophosphamide, methotrexate, 5-fluorouracil, vincristine

Table 10.5 The duration of adjuvant chemotherapy in randomized trials

Trial, (Reference) population	Investigated regimen	Investigated duration (months)	Relevant findings	Reported Results
Milan (Bonadonna et al, 1984)	CMF	6 vs 12	no difference	7 years
SAKK (Jungi et al, 1981)	oral LMF	6 vs 24	no difference	5 years
SECSG (Vélez-Garcia et al, 1984)				
(N+ 1–3)	CMF	6 vs 12	no difference	40 months
(N+ ≥4)	CMF (± RT)	6 (± RT) vs 12	no difference	40 months
SWOG (Rivkin et al, 1984b) (ER−)	CMFVP	12 vs 24	(ongoing) no difference	3 years
DFCI (Henderson et al, 1982) N+≥4 or high axillary N+	AC	5 vs 10*	no difference	6 years (median 2.5 years)

* 3- week cycles

Table 10.6 The timing of adjuvant chemotherapy administration in randomized trials

Trial, (Reference) population	Investigated treatments	Time of administration*	Reported follow-up	Relevant findings and Remarks
NSABP (Fisher et al, 1975a) pre. & post.	Thiotepa Control	days 0–2 (3 days)	10 years	Delay of recurrence specially in premenopausal patients with N+ ≥4
SACSG I (Nissen-Meyer et al, 1978) pre & post	C Control	days 0–5 (6 days)	15 years	RFS and OS advantage for treated patients A delay of treatment start resulted in disappearance of advantage
SACSG II (Nissen-Meyer et al, 1982)				
N−	− PeCT PeCT	days 0 + 7 days 0 + 7		No control group for N− population Trend of reduced relapses for the PeCT & ConCT as compared to PeCT alone
N+	PeCT + ConCT	days 0 + 7	4 years	
LBCS V (Ludwig Group, 1983)				
N−	PeCT Control	PeCT given within 36 h after mastectomy and again 7 days later	ongoing	Unpredictable and severe toxic effects resulted from possible interaction between nitrous oxide and methotrexate in the PeCT regimen; addition of Leucovorin rescue and more careful surveillance controlled severe toxic effects.
N+	PeCT PeCT + ConCT ConCT			
Cancer Research (Baum, 1982b) Campaign Adjuvant Trial	C C + T T	C as SACSG I T for 2 years	ongoing	PeCT with cyclophosphamide has been reported to be safe
Pre & post N−, N+	Control			

* Mastectomy on day O; C: Cyclophosphamid; T: Tamoxifen; PeCT: perioperative chemotherapy
ConCT: Conventionally-timed chemotherapy (start after removal of sutures).

and prednisone) was markedly diminished in patients who were treated with postoperative radiation and who did not receive chemotherapy until several weeks after the surgery. Buzdar et al (1982) reported on a series of patients with Stage II and III breast cancer treated with a FAC combination (5-fluorouracil, doxorubicin and cyclophosphamide) as adjuvant therapy. The length of time from surgery to initiation of FAC chemotherapy did not correlate with the length of disease-free survival in most subgroups. In subgroups with poor prognoses (Stage III patients) there was a suggestion that longer delays of chemotherapy were associated with shorter disease-free survival.

Adjuvant chemotherapy in patients without axillary lymph node metastasis

The axillary lymph node status has been described as the best prognostic indicator for survival in patients with operable carcinoma of the breast. At 10 years the failure rate for node-negative patients is 28%, with a 65% survival rate (Fisher et al, 1975a). A limited amount of data is available on treatment results in randomized prospective trials for patients properly staged and classified as having no metastasis in the axillary nodes. An early trial was reported (Kardinal & Donegan, 1980) in which patients were randomized to weekly thiotepa for one year or to no further therapy after mastectomy; this resulted in a long-term increase in relapse-free survival and overall survival in node-negative patients, especially those less than 55 years old. The OSAKO trial (Senn et al, 1984), in which 58 patients were treated with oral LMF (chlorambucil, methotrexate and 5-fluorouracil) and 68 received no further therapy after mastectomy, showed a statistically significant difference in overall survival between the two groups (p=0.02).

As the role of adjuvant chemotherapy in node-negative patients is not yet defined, the ongoing trials (Table 10.7) have a mastectomy-alone control group, even in 'high risk' subpopulations such as premenopausal patients with ER-negative tumors.

Adjuvant chemotherapy and the dose-response effect

The dose-response curve for most chemotherapeutic agents is steep (Frei E, 1980). When dose has been a randomized variable in clinical trials, a reproducible dose-response curve has generally been evident in leukemia, lymphoma, testicular cancer and small-cell lung cancer, all of which are highly sensitive to chemotherapy (Brindley, 1964; O'Bryan et al, 1977). In the adjuvant setting in breast cancer there is some evidence, based upon retrospective analysis, that dose is a factor in determining response. The results of adjuvant CMF therapy from Milan (Bonadonna & Valagussa, 1981) suggested a correlation between the dose received and the therapeutic effect

Table 10.7 Ongoing Randomized trials for node-negative breast cancer

Trial	Population	Design
ECOG 1180	ER+ and tumor size < 3 cm (pathol.)	— Registration only
	ER− or ER+ and tumor size ≥ 3 cm	{ CMFP × 6 Control
NSABP B-13	ER−	{ Sequential MTX/5FU/Leucovorin Control
Cancer Research Campaign Adjuvant Trial	all patients (N+ and N−)	{ C (PeCT) T × 2 years C (PeCT) + T × 2 years Control
LBCS V	all N−	{ PeCT CMF (2/3 of patients) Control (1/3 of patients)
Milan 8004	ER−	{ CMF × 12 cycles Control

PeCT	= perioperative chemotherapy	T	= Tamoxifen	F	= 5-fluorouracil
C	= cyclophosphamide	M	= methotrexate		

at 5 years follow-up. It seemed that the potential beneficial effect of adjuvant chemotherapy could have been obscured in postmenopausal patients because of dose reductions in women older than 60 years. Similar results were achieved in the OSAKO study (Senn et al, 1984) when a similar analysis was performed. In three other trials, the NSABP Melphalan vs Placebo Trial, the Guy's Hospital Melphalan vs Control and the LBCS III in which a mastectomy-alone control group was compared with a combination of chemo- and endocrine therapy, results failed to show any effect of dose (analyzed retrospectively) on outcome (Redmond et al, 1983; Rubens et al, 1983; Ludwig Breast Cancer Study Group, 1984).

No randomized trials comparing low and high doses of chemotherapy are being conducted at present. The dose-response relationship in various models and in the human cancers highly sensitive to chemotherapy would seem to have dissuaded most investigators from undertaking such an inquiry. Moreover, questions of toxicity and morbidity are in any case secondary to the more relevant, still unanswered, question of survival. Logic dictates that it is unlikely that a lower dose is more effective than a higher dose; therefore, the maximum dose possible should be delivered.

Conclusions

The various forms of adjuvant therapy investigated during the last three decades have produced some benefit. The following facts, however, could help to focus the problem of choosing a therapy outside a clinical trial.

(1) Adjuvant chemotherapy and endocrine therapy have resulted in a significant increase in relapse-free survival or disease-free survival, and some of

them, as well, in overall survival, during an observation period varying from 2–15 years after mastectomy in pre- and postmenopausal patients with axillary node involvement.

(2) Adjuvant combination chemotherapy is more effective than single-drug adjuvant treatment with melphalan alone.

(3) An intensive regimen using a five-drug combination might be more effective than a three-drug regimen in controlling disease. Definitive results from studies of treatments more intensive than the CMF regimen, with or without prednisone, are not yet available.

(4) Adjuvant chemotherapy might be more effective when given in the perioperative period; however, this must be confirmed by the results of ongoing trials involving early administration of adjuvant therapy.

The role of the combination of chemotherapy and endocrine therapy in the treatment of breast cancer is controversial.

The treatment of patients outside of trials

Premenopausal patients with 1–3 axillary node metastases should be treated with a CMF combination, while patients at higher risk for relapse (N+ ⩾4) should receive a more intensive combination chemotherapy. Recent information suggests that patients with ten or more positive axillary nodes may not benefit from any of the available combination chemotherapy regimens (Bonadonna et al, 1984, Fisher B et al, 1984).

For postmenopausal patients with axillary node involvement to whom it has been decided to administer adjuvant therapy, the choice between combined chemo- and endocrine therapy and endocrine therapy alone may be made on the basis of the steroid hormone receptor content of the primary breast tumor. No indication of an advantage from the addition of CMF to endocrine therapy (tamoxifen with or without prednisone) has emerged for patients with ER+ tumors. N+ patients with ER− tumors might benefit from an intensive five-drug combination chemotherapy (CMFVP).

Adjuvant therapy should not be administered to patients classified post-surgically as node-negative outside of the setting of clinical trials which have a mastectomy-alone control group. There is no definite evidence that the portion of this population with undetected systemic disease will benefit from adjuvant therapy, and the risk of overtreatment is significant in this patient population.

REFERENCES

Ahmann D L, Payne W S, Scanlon P W, O'Fallon J R, Bisel H F, Hahn R G et al 1978:
    Repeated adjuvant chemotherapy with phenylalanine mustard or 5-fluorouracil,
    cyclophosphamide and prednisone with or without radiation, after mastectomy for breast
    cancer. Lancet I: 893–896
Baum M 1982a Breast cancer—lessons from the past. Clinics in Oncology 3: 649–660
Baum M, Berstock D 1982b Breast cancer—adjuvant therapy. Clinics in Oncology 1: 901–915
BCTG/UICC/WHO 1984 Review of mortality results in randomized trials in early breast cancer.
    Lancet II: 1205
Boag J W, Haybittle J L, Powler J F, Emery E W 1971 The number of patients required in a
    clinical trial. British Journal of Radiology 44: 122–125

Bonadonna G, Valagussa P 1981 Dose-response effect of adjuvant chemotherapy in breast cancer. New England Journal of Medicine 30: 10–15

Bonadonna G, Rossi A, Tancini G, Brambilla C, Valagussa P 1984 Adjuvant chemotherapy trials in resectable breast cancer with positive axillary nodes. The experience of the Milan Cancer Institute. In Salmon S E, Jones S E (eds) Adjuvant Therapy of Cancer IV, Grune and Stratton, New York p 195–207

Brindley C O 1964 Further comparative trial of thio-phosphoro-amide and mechlorethamine in patients with melanoma and Hodgkin's disease. Journal of Chronic Diseases 17: 19–26

Buzdar A U, Smith T L, Powell K C, Blumenschein G T, Gehan E A 1981 Effect of timing of initiation of adjuvant chemotherapy on disease-free survival in breast cancer. Breast Cancer Research and Treatment 2: 163–169

Caprini J A, Oviedo M A, Cunningham M P, Cohen E, Trueheart R S, Khandekar J D, Scanlon E F 1980 Adjuvant chemotherapy for stage II and III breast carcinoma. Journal of the American Medical Association 244: 234–246

Carpenter J T, Maddox W A, Laws H L, Wirtschafter D D, Soong S J 1982 Favorable factors in the adjuvant therapy of breast cancer. Cancer 50: 18–23

Cooper M R, Rhyne A L, Muss H B, Ferree C, Richards, F, White D R et al 1981 A randomized comparative trial of chemotherapy and irradiation therapy for stage II breast cancer. Cancer 47: 2833–2839

Cooper R G, Holland J F, Glidewell O J 1979 Adjuvant chemotherapy of breast cancer. Cancer 44: 793–799

Creech R H, Dayal H, Alberts R, Catalano R B, Shah M K, Grotzinger P J 1983 A comparison of L-PAM and low-dose CMF as adjuvant therapy for breast cancer patients with nodal metastases. Proceedings of the American Association for Cancer Research 24:148

Davis H L, Metter G E, Ramirez G, Grage T B, Cornell G, Fletcher W et al 1979 An adjuvant trial of L-phenlyalanine mustard (L-PAM) versus cyclophosphamide (C), methotrexate (M), 5-fluorouracil (F) and vincristine (V)—CMF-V—following mastectomy for operable breast cancer. Proc American Society of Clinical Oncology 20:358

Fisher B, Slack N H, Katrych D, Wolmark N 1975a Ten years of follow-up results of patients with carcinoma of the breast in a cooperative clinical trial evaluating surgical adjuvant chemotherapy. Surgery, Gynaecology and Obstetrics 140: 528–534

Fisher B, Carbone P, Economou S G et al. 1975b L-phenylalanine mustard (L-PAM) in the management of primary breast cancer. A report of early findings. New England Journal of Medicine 292: 117–122

Fisher B, Redmond C, Fisher E R and participating NSABP investigators. 1980 The contribution of recent NSABP clinical trials of primary breast cancer therapy to an understanding of tumor biology—an overview of findings. Cancer 46: 1009–1025

Fisher B, Gunduz N, Saffer E A 1983a Influence of the interval between primary tumor removal and chemotherapy on kinetics and growth of metastases. Cancer Research 43: 1488–1492

Fisher B, Redmond C, Brown A, Wickerham D L, Wolkmark N, Allegra J et al 1983 Influence of tumor estrogen and progesterone receptor levels on the response to tamoxifen and chemotherapy in primary breast cancer. Journal of Clinical Oncology 4: 227–241

Fisher B, Redmond C, Fisher E R for NSABP 1984 A summary of findings from NSABP trials of adjuvant therapy. In: Salmon S E, Jones S E (eds) Adjuvant therapy of Cancer IV, Grune & Stratton, Florida p 185–194

Hellman S, Harris J R, Canellos G P, Fisher B 1982 Cancer of the breast. In: DeVitta V T, Hellman S, Rosenberg S A (eds) Cancer. Principles and practice of oncology. Lippincott, Philadelphia, p 914–970

Henderson I C, Gelman R, Parker L M, Skarin A T, Mayer R J Garnick M B et al 1982 15 vs 30 weeks of adjuvant chemotherapy for breast cancer patients with a high risk of recurrence: a randomized trial. Proceedings of the American Society for Clinical Oncology 1:75

Howat J M T, Hughes R, Durning P, George W D, Sellwood R A, Bush H et al 1981 A controlled clinical trial of adjuvant chemotherapy in operable cancer of the breast. In: Salmon S E, Jones S E (eds) Adjuvant therapy of cancer III. Grune & Stratton, New York p 371–376

Hubay C A, Pearson O H, Marshall J S, Stellato T A, Rhodes R S, DeBanne S M et al 1981 Adjuvant therapy of stage II breast cancer. Breast Cancer Research and Treatment 1: 77–82

Jungi W F, Alberto P, Brunner K W, Cavalli F, Barrelet L, Senn H J 1981 Short- or long-term adjuvant chemotherapy for breast cancer. In: Salmon S E, Jones S E (eds) Adjuvant Therapy of cancer III, Grune & Stratton, New York, p 395–402

Kardinal S G, Donegan W L 1980 Second cancers after prolonged adjuvant thiotepa for operable breast cancer. Cancer 45: 2042–2046

Ludwig Breast Cancer Study Group 1983 Toxic effects of early adjuvant chemotherapy for breast cancer. Lancet II: 542–544

Ludwig Breast Cancer Study Group 1984 Adjuvant therapy in postmenopausal women with operable breast cancer: Part I—A randomised trial of Chemo-Endocrine versus Endocrine Therapy versus mastectomy alone. In Salmon S E, Jones S E (eds) Adjuvant Therapy of cancer IV, Grune and Stratton, New York p 379–391

Morrison J M, Howell A, Grieve R J, Monypenny I H, Kelly K A, Marson A, Waterhouse J A, 1984 The West Midlands Oncology Association trials of Adjuvant Chemotherapy for operable breast cancer. In: Salmon S E and Jones S E (eds) Adjuvant Therapy of Cancer IV, Grune and Stratton, New York p 253–259

NIH 1980 Adjuvant chemotherapy of breast cancer. Summary of a NIH consensus statement. British Medical Journal 281: 724–725

Nissen-Meyer R, Kjellgren K, Malmio K, Mansson B, Norin T 1978 Surgical adjuvant chemotherapy. Results with one short course of cyclophosphamide after mastectomy for breast cancer. Cancer 41: 2088–2098

Nissen-Meyer R, Höst H, Kjellgren K, Mansson B, Norin T 1982 Perioperative adjuvant chemotherapy vs postoperatice chemotherapy for one year. Breast Cancer Research and Treatment 2: 391–394

O'Bryan R M, Baker L H, Gottlieb J E et al 1977 Dose-response evaluation of adriamycin in human neoplasia. Cancer 39: 1940–1948

Peto R 1982 Treatment of Cancer. Statistical aspects of cancer trials In: Treatment of Cancer Halnan K (eds) Wiend Chapman and Hall, London, p 867–871

Redmond C, Fisher B, Wiand H S 1983 The methodologic dilemma in retrospectively correlating the amount of chemotherapy received in adjuvant therapy protocols with disease-free survival. Cancer Treatment Reports 67: 519–526

Rivkin S E, Glucksberg H, Foulkes M 1984a Adjuvant chemotherapy for operable breast cancer with positive axillary nodes: A comparison of CMFVP versus L-Pam (South West Oncology Group Study) In: Salmon S E and Jones S E (eds) Adjuvant Therapy of Cancer IV. Grune and Stratton, New York p 209–215

Rivkin S E, Knight W A, Cruz A, Foulkes M, McDivitt R 1984b Adjuvant chemotherapy and hormonal therapy for operable breast cancer with positive axillary nodes. International Conference on the Adjuvant Therapy of Cancer, Tucson, Arizona, March

Rubens R D, Hayward J L, Knight R K et al 1983 Controlled trial of adjuvant chemotherapy with melphalan for breast cancer. Lancet I: 839–843

Senn H J, Jungi W F, for the OSAKO and SAKK groups 1984 Swiss adjuvant trials with LMF(+BCG) in N– and N+ Breast cancer. In: Salmon S E and Jones S E (eds) Adjuvant therapy of cancer IV, Grune and Stratton, New York p 261–270

Tormey D C, Weinberg V E, Holland J F et al 1983 A randomized trial of five- and three-drug chemotherapy and chemoimmuno-therapy in women with operable node-positive breast cancer. Journal of Clinical Oncology 1: 138–145

Tormey D C, Taylor S G, Kalish L A, Olson J E, Grage T, Gray R 1984 Adjuvant systemic therapy in premenopausal (CMF, CMFP, CMFPT) and postmenopausal (observation CMFP, CMFPT) women with node-positive breast cancer. In: Salmon S E and Jones S E (eds) Adjuvant therapy of Cancer IV, Grune and Stratton, New York, p. 359–368

Valagussa P, DiFronzo G, Bignami P, Buzzoni R, Bonadonna G, Veronesi U 1981 Prognostic importance of estrogen receptors to select node-negative patients for adjuvant chemotherapy. In: Salmon S E, Jones S E (eds) Adjuvant Therapy of Cancer III, Grune and Stratton, New York p 329–333

Vélez-Garcia E, Moore M, Vogel C L, Marcial V, Ketcham A, Raney M, Smalley R, 1984 Post surgical adjuvant chemotherapy with or without radiation therapy in women with breast cancer and positive capillary notes: The Southeastern Cancer Study Group (SECSG) experience. In: Salmon S E and Jones S E (eds) Adjuvant therapy of cancer IV, Grune and Stratton, New York p 273–282

Wheeler T K 1979 Four-drug combination chemotherapy following surgery for breast cancer. In: Salmon S E, Jones S E (eds) Adjuvant Therapy of Cancer II, Grune and Stratton, New York p 269–276

11 Practical management of patients with suspected breast cancer

JOHN S. SIMPSON

Introduction

It has been estimated that 25% of women will seek medical advice for a breast abnormality at some time in their lives (Townsend, 1980). It is clear that for many of these women the prime fear is a diagnosis of breast cancer. Between 4.4% (Mahoney, 1977) and 13% (Devitt, 1977) of the women attending a breast clinic will be found to have breast cancer. It can be seen from these figures that breast pathology is common and that there is a real risk that a woman with a breast abnormality could have cancer. A clinician managing breast problems must be able to make an accurate assessment as to whether or not a particular patient has malignant breast disease. This diagnostic process should take place as rapidly as possible in order to limit the duration of the enormous emotional burden borne by many patients. There is no clear consensus about how the diagnostic phase of management should be conducted and the clinician is faced with a wide range of different options for investigation and biopsy. Likewise, the surgeon must decide between a number of different operations for the definitive treatment of established breast cancer. This subject has often produced lively debate and the recent increase in interest in alternatives to mastectomy has rekindled the debate. The practical management from presentation to definitive surgery may be considered in four phases (Fig. 11.1).

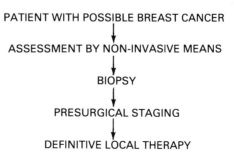

Fig. 11.1 Sequence of management

Assessment by non-invasive methods

The traditional method of managing breast abnormalities has consisted of only clinical evaluation for pre-operative assessment. Following such assessment, standard practice has been to perform open surgical biopsy on a high proportion of patients with a palpable abnormality. This management philosophy is summarized by the maxim 'a lump is better out than in'. Such a policy may be expected to have a high true positive rate but will also result in the performance of many biopsies for non-malignant conditions. In the last 30 years, a wide range of new methods for the investigation of women with breast abnormalities has been developed. Such developments have added greatly to the complexity but also to the accuracy of pre-operative assessment. The aim must be to use this technology to achieve the highest possible true positive and true negative rates for the diagnostic process. Non-invasive methods used at the present time include clinical assessment, mammography, galactography, ultrasound, CT scanning, thermography, diaphanography and magnetic resonance imaging.

Clinical assessment

Predictably, there have been no startling recent advances in the area of clinical diagnosis. However, there have been a number of interesting reports about the presentation of breast cancer which contribute to the planning of clinical assessment. The great majority of women present with a breast mass but a small number present with pain. Mastalgia alone may be the presenting symptom in 5% (Yorkshire Breast Cancer Group, 1983) to 7% per cent (Preece et al, 1982) of carcinomas.

The value of a detailed, time-consuming, clinical history has been questioned and the suggestion made that only the patient's age and family history are important in increasing the suspicion of malignant disease (Devitt, 1977). The same author (Devitt, 1983) has emphasised the importance of inspection in examination of the breast and found that 69% of patients with cancer had a visable abnormality such as dimpling.

Mammography

Mammography has had an established place in the diagnosis of breast cancer since the first large series reporting its use was published in 1960 (Egan, 1960). It has been used both as a diagnostic aid in symptomatic patients and as a means of screening those without symptoms. The importance of the screening role for mammography has been demonstrated in two large American studies, the Health Insurance Plan (HIP) study (Strax et al, 1973) and the Breast Cancer Demonstration Detection Project (BCDDP) study (Baker, 1982). The BCDDP study, in particular, indicates the importance of mammography, as a screening modality. Mammography detected a significant proportion of cancers (41.6%) which were not detected by clinical means. Population screening by mammography may well lead to a reduced mortality from breast cancer but the cost of making screening available generally is too great for all but the most affluent societies.

In the early days of mammography there were fears about possible carcinogenic effects of the radiation received by the breast. These fears have been removed to a great extent by advances in machine and film technology. With the use of contemporary equipment the radiation dose per examination is likely to be 2.5–5 mGy rads. This represents at least a ten-fold reduction in radiation dose compared with the early days of mammography and means that even multiple examinations are very unlikely to be harmful (Feig, 1984).

In symptomatic women with possible breast cancer, mammography is commonly used as a routine part of the diagnostic process. In many clinics, a lower age limit of 30 or 35 years is employed for routine use. Below this age, the prevalence of breast cancer makes a positive result unlikely and small malignant lesions are likely to be obscured by the dense dysplastic breast tissue found in younger women. In addition to providing diagnostic information about a possible cancer, mammography also can detect impalpable and perhaps unsuspected cancers. It can demonstrate multifocal disease in the same or contralateral breast.

Information about the presence or absence of multifocal disease is of particular importance when surgical biopsy is being planned and when breast conserving surgery is being considered. In addition mammography of the contralateral breast provides a baseline for follow-up examinations to detect second primary tumours.

Mammography has been shown to be a more accurate diagnostic test than clinical examination or a range of alternative tests (Table 11.1). Only computerized tomography has been shown to be more accurate (Chang et al, 1980). Despite this, the problem of cancers missed by mammography is an important one (Martin et al, 1979). Reasons given for missed diagnoses are:
(a) Poor radiographic technique
(b) Obvious oversight by the radiologist
(c) Failure to recognise subtle radiographic signs
(d) Real absence of the radiographic criteria of cancer.

An apparently normal mammogram, should not be used, on its own, to exclude cancer and management should be planned when the results of clinical

Table 11.1 Accuracy of diagnostic tests

Method	Author	No. of Cases	True Positive Rate	False Positive Rate
Mammography	Egan et al (1977)	1003	87%	6%
	Dodd (1977)	65 000 (Collected Series)	87.2%	14.9%
CT Scanning	Chang (1980, 1982)	1625	94%	—
Thermography	Byrne & Yerex (1975)	2275	81%	32%
	Isard et al (1972)	10 055	71%	28%
	Sterns et al (1982)	502	36%	6.4–11.7%*
	Lapayowker & Revesz (1980)	44 525 (Collected Series)	72%	23%
Ultrasonography	Dodd (1977)	—	86%	—

* Two methods used

assessment and other investigations have been considered. If there is any degree of clinical suspicion serious consideration should be given to some form of biopsy.

False positive results can also lead to considerable anxiety and to unnecessary surgery. The prospects of such a false positive result are high when mammographic microcalcifications are the only abnormality. Powell et al (1983) have reported a series of these abnormalities in which only 17% of the biopsies were malignant. The most helpful finding from Powell's study was that a minimum of five separate grains should be present for an abnormality to qualify as an area of suspicious microcalcification. However, it is not easy to distinguish between benign and malignant microcalcifications (Colbassani et al, 1982). A recently described cause of a false positive result is a haematoma following fine needle aspiration (Sickles et al, 1983a). The authors recommend an interval of at least 2 weeks between aspiration and mammography.

Galactography
This technique has been recommended as the investigation of choice in women with a serous or bloody nipple discharge (Tabar et al, 1983). Cannulation of the offending lactiferous duct is performed and the duct system is then injected with water soluble contrast. This test is comparatively little used but appears to be a more accurate method of confirming the presence of a carcinoma than either mammography or cytological examination of the discharge.

Computerized tomography
The development of whole-body computerized tomography (CT) in the 1970s has led to the use of the scanner for breast imaging. Chang et al (1980) have reported the use of a dedicated breast scanner and also the use of a standard body scanner (Chang et al, 1982). The dedicated scanner, which uses a water immersion technique, gives an average radiation dose of 1.75 mGy rads per examination. The technique includes contrast medium enhancement with diatrizoate meglumine, an iodide compound. The iodide is taken up selectively by tumour tissue and this is reflected in the CT number obtained. The authors claim that the use of CT with contrast enchancement adds a further dimension to breast imaging and enables small cancers to be detected in dense dysplastic breasts. The true positivity rate for breast CT (94%) is higher than for film mammography (77%) (Chang et al, 1980). Whether the high capital cost of a dedicated breast scanner will ever be justified by improved results, remains to be seen.

Ultrasound
This method of breast imaging is free from any concern about radiation effects and appears to be completely safe. It is used either with a water immersion technique or by the contact real-time method. Both methods reliably distinguish solid from cystic masses. The resolution of ultrasound is such that 1 cm lesions should be detected without difficulty and it may detect lesions as small as 5 mm. Sonography can play an important role in the management of small lesions identified by mammography. By clearly identifying certain lesions as cysts unnecessary biopsies can be avoided (Teixidor, 1980). It is, however,

less successful than mammography in making the distinction between benign and malignant solid lesions. (Sickles et al, 1983b). Fibroadenomas, by virtue of the presence of smooth walls, are readily identified by ultrasound and it may have a useful diagnostic role in young patients for whom mammography is inappropriate. However, its most valuable role seems to be as an adjunct to mammography rather than as a diagnostic or screening technique in its own right.

Thermogprahy
This method of breast cancer detection, like ultrasonography, avoids radiation exposure and also appears free of hazard to the patient. Thermal patterns over the breast can be detected in a number of ways, for example, infra-red thermography, micro-wave thermography or liquid crystal or plate thermography. In addition to its diagnostic role thermography has been advocated as a means of selecting women for mammography and as a means of predicting future risk of breast cancer (Gautherie & Gros, 1980). The overwhelming impression now is that the diagnostic accuracy of the method is too low to be of real value (Sterns et al, 1982). Both high false negative and false positive rates are a feature of most published series using thermography (Dodd, 1977). It was included in the original protocol for the BCDDP screening programme but was dropped in 1976 when a false negative rate of almost 50% was found in women with proven breast cancer. The rate is even higher for lesions of 1 cm or less. As the presence of an abnormal thermal pattern appears to be a function of both the size and the biology of the tumour, thermography appears to be of little use in detecting small, potentially curable, cancers. Also, it seems unlikely to be useful in selecting women for mammographic screening.

Diaphanography
This is another non-invasive technique which employs transillumination of the breast, in a darkened room, to detect abnormalities (Watmough, 1983). It is associated with high false negative rates in all but the largest tumours and requires complex technology for image recording. It probably has no diagnostic role.

Magnetic resonance imaging
This is a new addition to the methods for breast imaging which appears to offer real promise. It uses electro-magnetic waves and appears to be entirely safe. As yet there are no reports of its accuracy in the diagnosis of breast cancer.

Biopsy options

A tissue diagnosis to confirm the presence of breast cancer is essential before definitive surgery is performed. In the past, open biopsy was the only option, but now the choice lies between open biopsy, core needle biopsy and fine needle aspiration. Each of these methods has important advantages and disadvantages which are summarized in Table 11.2.

Table 11.2 Comparison of biopsy methods

	Clinic Procedure	Well tolerated by patient	Suitable small tumours	Suitable large tumours	High True +ve	Low False +ve
Open biopsy GA	—	+	+++	+++	+++	+++
Open biopsy LA	+/−	++	+++	+	+++	+++
Trucut core or drill biopsy	+++	++	+/−	+++	++	+++
Fine needle aspiration	+++	+++	+	+++	++	++

Open biopsy

This includes incision or excision biopsy of the tumour performed under general or local anaesthesia. A specimen of tissue is obtained for histopathological assessment and for hormone receptor and other assays requiring tumour tissue. A full histological evaluation of this type of specimen is most unlikely to produce either false positive or false negative results. In particular, the sort of sampling error which is associated with needle biopsy is a very rare event.

Immediate reporting of open biopsies can be achieved by the use of frozen section preparations of the tumour tissue (Bauermeister, 1980). There is a very high correlation between the results of a frozen section examination and the final histopathology report. At times there may be a real difficulty in reaching a decision on frozen section material. There is clearly a place for the pathologist to give a verdict of 'uncertain' on the frozen section and delay a final decision until permanent sections have been examined.

Frozen section examinations have been used for many years to obtain a tissue diagnosis prior to performing a mastectomy under the same anaesthetic. This process sometimes known as the 'one-stage' procedure has been the subject of much discussion in recent years and was regarded as undesirable by a Consensus Development Conference in the United States (Moxley et al, 1980). There is a strong body of opinion that the biopsy to obtain a tissue diagnosis and the mastectomy should be performed as separate operations (two-stage procedure). This enables the patient to have time to consider and discuss treatment options in the light of a definite diagnosis of cancer. It has been suggested that the two-stage procedure might be associated with less psychosocial morbidity but, as yet, there is no evidence to confirm this view (Maguire & Van Dam, 1983). A recent study in Wellington, New Zealand suggested that older women prefer a one-state procedure while younger women (under 50) are more inclined to choose a two-stage operation (Simpson, 1984). It seems likely that allowing the woman to decide which type of procedure she has could be the answer to this problem.

A further important role for frozen section examinations is to provide an immediate reliable biopsy result even when no further surgery is planned under the same anaesthetic. This allows the patient to be given the diagnosis at the first possible opportunity and it enables arrangements to be made for investigations and further management.

Biopsy under local anaesthesia

When breast biopsy is performed under local anaesthesia it can usually be done on an out-patient basis whereas biopsy under general anaesthesia commonly requires hospital admission. Hospital stay is longer when general anaesthesia is used, greater expense is incurred and there is some additional morbidity. Biopsy under local anaesthesia is well accepted by almost all patients (Walker et al, 1978) and is suitable for excision of all but the largest and deepest breast lumps. With suitable preliminary sedation and by adequate use of a local anaesthetic agent containing adrenaline, it is rarely a significantly distressing or uncomfortable procedure.

Core needle biopsy

A core of tissue for histological examination can be obtained without difficulty using a Trucut biopsy needle (Travenol Laboratories) or by drill biopsy using a high speed compressed-air drill. The air drill (Meyerowitz et al, 1965) obtains a satisfactory specimen of tissue but the noise of the drill can be disturbing. Trucut biopsy is a reliable method of obtaining tissue for histopathology (Roberts et al, 1975). The technique of performing a Trucut biopsy is easily learnt and is facilitated by using a Pistomat pistol-grip handle (Brun del Re, 1979). This device enables the tumour to be held in one hand while the biopsy needle is operated without difficulty with the other.

False positive results are not a feature of this technique but false negative findings may result from sampling error or from failure to obtain a core of very hard tumour tissue. The accuracy of Trucut biopsy (Table 11.3) increases with tumour size (Roberts et al, 1975). Sampling error becomes a major problem in masses less than 2 cm in diameter and open biopsy is usually preferable for such tumours. The technique is generally well tolerated but some apprehension and pain are common despite the use of local anaesthesia.

Fine needle aspiration (FNA)

This technique of obtaining material from breast lumps for cytological examination has been widely used in Sweden for many years (Franzen & Zajicek, 1968). Its acceptance in many other countries has come more recently (Straw-

Table 11.3 Accuracy of trucut core and drill biopsy

	No. of cases	True positive rate	False positive rate
Shabot et al (1981)[*]	81	78.9%	0%
Davies et al (1977)[*]	131	74%	0%
Roberts et al (1975)[*]	203	70%	0%
Dowle and Simpson (1984)[*]	135	83%	0%
George and Burn (1975)[+]	1720	85%	0%
Meyerowitz (1976)[+]	135	98.5%	0%

[*] —Trucut biopsy
[+] —drill biopsy

Table 11.4 Fine needle aspiration

Author	No. of cases	True positive rate*	false positive rate*
Rimsten et al (1975)	984	82.5%	0.2%
Davies et al (1977)	131	52%	14.3%
Kline et al (1979)	3545	90.5%	1.89%
Duguid et al (1979)	294	93.3%	7.7%
Strawbridge et al (1981)	3724	69.5%	4.4%
Bell et al (1983)	1410	72.1%	6.2%

* These rates have been recalculated to give comparable figures

bridge et al, 1981). It has the important advantages over other biopsy techniques of being cheap, easy to perform, well accepted by patients and virtually free of complications (Table 11.2). When used in an institution with good coordination between cytopathologist and surgeon it provides a highly accurate means of obtaining a tissue diagnosis (Bell et al, 1983). A very high true positive and a zero false positive rate can be expected under these circumstances (Table 11.4). However, false positive results have been reported (Davies et al, 1977) and are of great concern. It is essential that any clinic or institution should evaluate its own results carefully before using FNA as the basis for performing definitive surgery (Abele et al, 1983). Until it is clear that the probability of a false positive result is effective zero, a 'malignant' FNA result should not be used as the basis for definitive surgery. Under these circumstances a core needle or open biopsy should follow the FNA as shown in the diagnostic plan (Fig. 11.2).

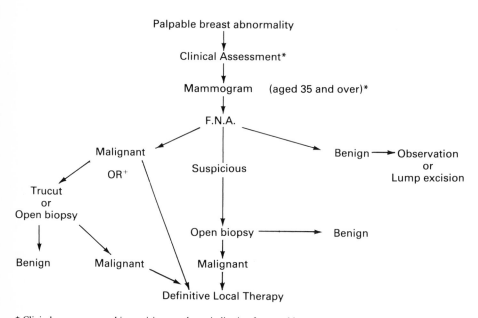

* Clinical or mammographic suspicion may be an indication for open biopsy
+ Depending on whether or not FNA has been accepted as the basis for definitive therapy

Fig. 11.2 Diagnostic algorithm

Pre-surgical staging

If biopsy and definitive surgery are carried out independently (two-stage procedure), there is an opportunity to perform investigations, between the two operations, which will define the patient's overall disease status. A tissue diagnosis of breast cancer can then be followed by pre-surgical staging of possible metastatic disease sites. If a one-stage procedure is used such investigations must either be performed before a certain diagnosis of cancer is made or postponed until after mastectomy or other definitive surgical procedure. If staging investigations are performed after mastectomy it is obvious that surgical management cannot be influenced by the results. However if occult metastatic disease is detected prior to definitive surgery the whole management plan is likely to be altered radically. The disease is then almost certainly incurable and the only possible reason for performing mastectomy will be for the control of local disease. The emphasis in management will then be directed towards systemic therapy and the use of mastectomy is only likely to increase psychosocial morbidity in an already difficult situation.

A positive result from a staging investigation is therefore of considerable management importance and the value of a particular test in this context must depend on the probability of such a result. The common sites for distant metastases in breast cancer are: bone, liver, lung and brain and the value of investigations to 'stage' each of these sites will be considered.

Bone metastases

Breast cancer commonly forms metastases in the skeleton and these can readily be demonstrated scintigraphically using ^{99m}Tc phosphate compounds. This technique enables the whole skeleton to be examined rapidly and is capable of greater resolution than conventional skeletal radiology. It is non-specific in that local increases in isotope uptake ('hot spots') can be due to a variety of bone conditions associated with new bone formation, such as healing fractures. It is essential, therefore, that 'hot-spots' on the scan should be investigated further by bone X-rays. By this method, three separate groups of patients with a bone scan abnormality can be identified

(a) Those with normal X-rays of the 'hot spot'

(b) Those with a benign abnormality at the same site

(c) Those with a radiological abnormality suggestive of metastatic disease.

If a scan abnormality is accompanied by the appearances of metastatic disease radiologically, there can be no reasonable doubt. Likewise a benign abnormality on X-ray is likely to be accepted as the explanation for the 'hot spot'. This leaves a group of 27% of patients with abnormal scans whose X-rays are normal (Citrin et al, 1975). When the abnormal scan is the only positive result management decisions are difficult since many, but not all, patients in this situation go on to develop overt bone disease (Campbell et al, 1976). A suggested working rule is to regard one or two single unexplained 'hot spots' as suspicious but not diagnostic and multiple 'hot spots' as diagnostic of bone metastases. Bone biopsy, if this can be done, is of considerable value in the case of an unexplained 'hot-spot'. The use of computerized tomography also may help to resolve a number of problems of this type.

Bone scanning prior to definitive surgery has been widely advocated on the grounds that a positive result will lead to a major change in management policy (Campbell et al, 1976). The policy has been challenged on the grounds that the low abnormality rate makes the investigation non cost-effective (Lee, 1981). In a series of published reports summarized by Lee, the rate of positive bone scans ranged from 4% to 45% for all patients presenting with breast cancer, with a median of 11%. When only clinical stage I and II cancers are considered the range is 1–40 per cent with a median of 6%. Positivity is related to tumour size with a very low rate in T_1 tumours, low in T_2 tumours and only in T_3 tumours does the rate exceed 10% (McNeil et al, 1978). The reported incidence of positive scans (Table 11.5) is lower in the more recently reported series and this may be explained by changes in the breast cancer population or by technological improvements which reduce the false positive rate. Despite these doubts bone scanning remains the pre-operative staging investigation which is most likely to be positive and hence alter management. Although the chances of a positive result are small the impact on management is great and the scan will serve as a base-line for future investigations. There must still be a strong case for its routine use.

Table 11.5 Bone scanning in 'early' breast cancer

Author	No. of Patients	Isotope used	Total % Positive	Tumour size		
				T_1	T_2	T_3
Galasko (1975)	50	18F	24%	—	—	—
El-Domeiri & Shroff (1976)	55	^{99m}Tc	27%	0%	8%	40%
Clark et al (1978)	201	^{99m}Tc	11%	7%*	4%*	39%*
O'Connell et al (1978)	85	^{99m}Tc	6%	3%+	9%+	0%+
McNeil et al (1978)	153	^{99m}Tc	7%	0%	6%	19%
British Breast Group (1978)	994 (collected series)	^{99m}Tc	10%	—	—	—
Total	1538		11%			

* TNM staging
+ Pathological staging

Conventional bone marrow examination by cytological means has been suggested as a means of verifying the presence of metastases in a patient with a positive bone scan (Landys, 1982). It is most unlikely to be of value in bone scan negative patients except perhaps in those with locally more advanced disease. The use of radiolabelled monoclonal antibodies to label malignant cells in the marrow (Rainsbury et al, 1983; Redding et al, 1983) had dramatically altered the potential value of marrow examination. Tumour cells have been detected by the use of a breast epithelial monoclonal antibody in 28% of patients with primary breast cancer. None were detected by conventional marrow examination and scintigraphy was normal. This investigation, if validated, may prove to be the most valuable of all pre-surgical staging investigations and could supersede bone scanning in many instances.

Liver metastases

Imaging of the liver in patients with operable breast cancer is an unrewarding process. The use of liver scanning with ^{99m}Tc sulphur colloid is likely to produce a true positive rate of less than 1% when liver disease is not otherwise suspected (Weiner & Sachs, 1978). This technique is generally associated with a high rate of false positive and false negative results and seems of little value as a staging investigation. Computerized tomography (CT) and ultrasonography have been compared with scintigraphy in patients with breast and colon cancer (Alderson et al, 1983). Alderson concluded that scintigraphy was the most valuable liver imaging investigation in breast cancer although he found that CT was better for investigating colon cancer. Liver function tests are readily and cheaply performed in all hospitals and, although associated with a high false positive rate, are valuable in terms of a high true positive rate. A reasonable policy for pre-surgical staging is to perform routinely liver function tests (SGOT, SGPT, GGT and alkaline phosphatase) and to base requests for further imaging by scintigraphy or CT on the results of these tests.

Brain metastases

It is common for patients to have cerebral metastases at the time of death but it is rare for these to be detectable in asymptomatic patients. Both scintigraphic brain scanning and computerized tomography are remotely unlikely to detect otherwise unsuspected brain metastases even when the primary breast tumour is locally advanced (Lewi et al, 1980). Brain imaging is therefore not recommended as a pre-surgical staging investigation.

Lung metastases

A single exposure chest X-ray is a standard part of the pre-operative work-up and may very occasionally detect an asymptomatic pulmonary metastasis. There is no evidence to suggest that additional investigations such as conventional lung tomography or computerized tomography can be justified as a routine part of the staging process.

Local therapy

The choice of options for the management of local disease in breast cancer is now wider and more confusing than ever before (Table 11.6). Total mastectomy and axillary dissection has been identified by the Consensus Development Conference as 'standard therapy' (Moxley et al, 1980), but a number of recent reports have led to increasing use, in selected patients, of

Table 11.6 Options for definitive local therapy

RADIOTHERAPY ALONE
WIDE LOCAL EXCISION ALONE
WIDE LOCAL EXCISION AND RADIOTHERAPY
TOTAL MASTECTOMY AND AXILLARY DISSECTION

wide local excision and radiotherapy (Veronesi et al, 1981) and radiotherapy alone (Harris et al, 1978). The rationale for using these alternatives to mastectomy and their advantages and disadvantages is beyond the scope of this chapter and only mastectomy will be discussed here.

Ideas about the metastatic process in breast cancer have changed markedly since the use of the radical mastectomy was first reported by Halsted in 1894. Breast cancer was believed to spread sequentially from its local origins in the breast, to regional lymph nodes and finally to distant sites. If the surgical procedure was performed early enough in the natural history of the disease and was sufficiently radical, cure would result. This concept of spread of the disease resulted in first the radical mastectomy and later the extended radical and other more extensive surgical procedures. These major resections sought to achieve cure by wide excision of all involved lymph nodes. Clinical trials have failed to demonstrate any improvement in survival with increasing scope of the nodal resection (Veronesi & Valagussa, 1981).

When attempts to alter the natural history of the disease by more radical surgery failed, a new theory for tumour spread evolved. This may be termed the 'systemic disease from the outset' hypothesis which explains treatment failure on the grounds that the disease is always systemic (Fisher, 1977). Hence it is unlikely that variations in local therapy will be of major significance and nodal involvement is an expression of the tumour/host relationship rather than as a definite stage in the spread of the disease. In accepting the systemic disease hypothesis the rationale for the Halsted radical mastectomy becomes no longer acceptable. Thus in continuing to perform mastectomy, albeit not Halsted's operation, we must consider carefully what is the justification for the continuing use of this procedure.

The rationale for mastectomy in the 1980s
In rejecting the traditional hypothesis for disease spread we must be careful to replace it with one that is plausible for today's clinicians. The 'systemic disease from the outset' theory leads to the conclusion that differences in primary therapy will have no effect on prognosis. It also follows that the value of early diagnosis and hence early surgery must be questioned. If these conclusions about primary therapy were accepted attempts at early diagnosis by the methods outlined in this chapter would appear futile and the continued use of mastectomy could not be justified.

Breast cancer is a heterogeneous disease and from clinical observations of its natural history it seems likely that a small minority of tumours spread in a sequential fashion and it also seems probable that in another proportion metastatic disease is present from the outset. It is conceivable that for many tumours an element of both types of behaviour is apparent at different stages in the malignant process. The disease may well be confined to the breast for the first part of its natural history after which dissemination occurs. Host defence factors probably have a profound influence on the timing of this dissemination. Metastases will develop in distant sites in most patients but in some patients they may be confined, for a time, to regional lymph nodes. If this model of spread is accurate, local therapy will be of considerable importance for the 'early' tumour confined to the breast and for those tumours that have spread to regional lymph nodes but not to distant sites.

It is likely, however, that the great majority of patients will have a predetermined outcome at the time of presentation and therefore variations in local therapy are not likely to affect their outcome. Once distant metastases are established it seems most unlikely that primary therapy will have a major influence on prognosis although removal of the primary may modify the growth kinetics of the secondary tumour. Since precise identification of which tumours are localized is not yet possible, a surgical strategy must be developed which will deal effectively with localized tumours. In this way the prospect of offering some patients curative therapy by surgical means will not be lost.

Potentially curative surgery for the supposedly localized tumour would consist of
(a) Complete removal of the primary tumour
(b) Removal of any multifocal disease in the same breast
(c) Removal of lymphatic and venous channels containing tumour cells.
The case for total excision of breast tissue rests on the inability of breast-conserving surgery to ensure that these three aims are achieved. Perhaps the most uncertain entity of the three is multifocal disease. Its true incidence is debatable with reported rates ranging from less than 10% to more than 30 per cent. When a simulated partial mastectomy (excision of a quadrant of the breast on a mastectomy specimen) was performed on different types of breast cancer, residual tumour was found in the remaining breast tissue in 26% of patients with T_1 tumours, in 38% of T_2 or T_3 tumours and in 80% of sub-areolar tumours (Rosen et al, 1975). Many of these multifocal tumours are pre-invasive but nonetheless there is real concern about eventual invasive tumour development. Clearly this concern can be removed by total mastectomy.

The case for axillary dissection as an essential ingredient of primary surgical treatment rests on three quite separate considerations. These are:
(a) The need to examine axillary lymph nodes as a means of assessing prognosis
(b) Reduction of the risk of unpleasant progressive regional disease
(c) To influence survival in a small number of patients.
There is good evidence that the number of nodes involved (Fisher et al, 1983) and nodal status i.e. no involved nodes, 1–3 or 4 plus involved nodes provides a good indication of prognosis (Fisher et al, 1975). This prognostic information is widely used in decision making about adjuvant therapy.

Patient acceptability is now a major factor in the choice of local therapy. No woman finds a mastectomy anything but distressing but the distress can be minimized by efforts to achieve a satisfactory cosmetic and functional result. There is no evidence that resection of pectoralis major improves survival and there is clear evidence that visible ribs and shoulder weakness are unpleasant consequences. There would seem to be few instances where pectoralis major should be excised. Likewise a low horizontal scar is likely to be more acceptable than one that is visible above clothing. These considerations are important to the patient and are compatible with the commonly used techniques for total mastectomy and axillary dissection (sometimes called modified radical mastectomy).

Clinical trials of mastectomy

Many randomized clinical trials have been conducted over the years comparing one type of primary procedure with others. In addition numerous non-controlled series have been reported. A selection of both types of report are summarized in Table 11.7. Halsted mastectomy has been compared with more radical procedures and no difference in survival shown (Veronesi & Valagussa, 1981; Kaae & Johansen, 1968). When the Halsted mastectomy has been compared with less radical procedures again no survival differences have been shown. Modified radical mastectomy has been shown to give comparable survival with radical mastectomy in a number of studies, one of which revealed a higher local recurrence rate in the modified radical group (Maddock et al, 1982). Radical mastectomy has been shown to be equivalent to simple mastectomy followed by radiotherapy (Hamilton et al, 1974). The latter policy has, in turn, been shown to give similar survival to simple mastectomy alone although the radiotherapy group did have a significantly lower incidence of local recurrence (Cancer Research Campaign Working Party 1980). Overall there is a remarkable similarity of survival at 5 and 10 years (Table 11.7).

Table 11.7 Prognosis after mastectomy for 'Operable' breast cancer

	Author	No. of patients	patients randomized	Survival 5 yrs	10 yrs
Halsted radical	Fisher et al (1975)	406	Yes	64%	46%
	Turner et al (1981)	278	Yes	70%	
	Veronesi and Costa (1982)	372	Yes	—	50%
Extended radical	Kaae & Johansen (1968)	271	Yes	65%	44%
	Veronesi and Costa (1982)	344	Yes	—	47%
Modified radical	Leis (1980)	564	No	—	63%
	Turner et al (1981)	256	Yes	70%	—
Simple & Radiotherapy	Cancer Research Campaign (1980)	1103	Yes	73%	—
	Kaae and Johansen (1968)	288	Yes	62%	42%
Simple alone	Cancer Research Campaign (1980)	1140	Yes	70%	—

Rehabilitation

Mastectomy has been known to be associated with both physical and psychological problems. The physical problems after mastectomy include shoulder stiffness, arm weakness and oedema and abnormal upper arm and chest wall sensation. With the type of surgery described, followed by an active rehabilitation programme, long term problems should be rare and minor.

Of much greater concern is the prospect of psychosocial morbidity. This is common and at times severe (Morris, 1983). Depression and sexual difficulties occur in 25–30% of patients (Maguire et al, 1978) in the first year after mastectomy. Those at particular risk include women with past or present psychiatric problems, those without good support and the unemployed. The use of specialized nursing support, counselling, volunteer groups and a readiness to seek psychiatric help, all contribute to minimizing these problems.

Reconstruction after mastectomy

Part of the morbidity of the management sequence, which includes mastectomy, is directly related to breast loss. This effect can be overcome to a considerable extent by the use of breast reconstruction procedures. This can be carried out by means of a synthetic implant and/or the use of a latissimus dorsi flap (Hughes & Webster, 1981). Reconstruction can be performed at the time of mastectomy (Nash & Hurst, 1982) or at any time thereafter. A study from Edinburgh has shown that immediate reconstruction is helpful in avoiding some psychiatric morbidity (Dean et al, 1983).

REFERENCES

Abele J S, Miller T R, Goodson W H III, Hunt T K, Hohn D C 1983 Fine-needle aspiration of palpable breast masses. A programme for staged implementation. Archives of Surgery 118: 859–863
Alderson P O, Adams D F, McNeil B J, Sanders R, Siegelman S S, Finberg H J et al 1983 Computed tomography, ultrasound, and scintigraphy of the liver in patients with colon or breast carcinoma: a prospective comparison. Radiology 149: 225–230
Baker L H 1982 Breast cancer detection demonstration project: five-year summary report. CA-A Cancer Journal for Clinicians 32: 194–225
Bauermeister D E 1980 The role and limitations of frozen section and needle aspiration biopsy in breast cancer diagnosis. Cancer 46: 947–949
Bell D A, Hajdu S I, Urban J A, Gaston J P 1983 Role of aspiration cytology in the diagnosis and management of mammary lesions in office practice. Cancer 51: 1182–1189
British Breast Group 1978 Bone scanning in breast cancer. British Medical Journal 2: 180–181
Brun del Re R 1980 A new spring-loaded biopsy handle for improved needle biopsy. British Journal of Surgery 67: 449–450
Byrne R R, Yerex J A 1975 The three roles of breast thermography. Applied Radiology 4: 53–58
Campbell D J, Banks A J, Oates G D 1976 The value of preliminary bone scanning in staging and assessing the prognosis of breast cancer. British Journal of Surgery 63: 811–816
Cancer Research Campaign Working Party 1980 Cancer research campaign trial for early breast cancer. Lancet II: 55–60
Chang C H J, Sibala J L, Fritz S L, Dwyer S J III, Templeton A W, Lin F et al 1980 Computed tomography in detection and diagnosis of breast cancer. Cancer 46: 939–946
Chang C H J, Nesbit D E, Fisher D R, Fritz S L, Dwyer S J III, Templeton A W et al 1982 Computed tomographic mammography using a conventional body scanner. American Journal of Roentgenology 138: 553–558
Citrin D L, Bessent R G, Greig W R, McKellar N J, Furnival C, Blumgart L H 1975 The application of the ^{99m}Tc phosphate bone scan to the study of breast cancer. British Journal of Surgery 62: 201–204
Clark D G, Painter R W, Sziklas J J 1978 Indications for bone scans in preoperative evaluation of breast cancer. American Journal of Surgery 135: 667–670
Colbassani H J, Feller W F, Cigtay O S, Chun B 1982 Mammographic and pathological correlation of microcalcification in disease of the breast. Surgery, Gynecology and Obstetrics 155: 689–696

Davies C J, Elston C W, Cotton R E, Blamey R W 1977 Preoperative diagnosis in carcinoma of the breast. British Journal of Surgery 64: 326–328

Dean C, Chetty U, Forrest A P M 1983 Effects of immediate breast reconstruction on psychosocial morbidity after mastectomy. Lancet I: 459–462

Devitt J E 1977 Value of the history in the office diagnosis of breast cancer. Canadian Medical Association Journal 116: 1127–1128

Devitt J E 1983 How breast cancer presents. Canadian Medical Association Journal 129: 43–47

Dodd G D 1977 Present status of thermography, ultrasound and mammography in breast cancer detection. Cancer 39: 2796–2805

Dowle C, Simpson J S 1984 Trucut biopsy for breast cancer, factors influencing accuracy (In preparation)

Duguid H L, Wood R A B, Irving A D, Preece P E, Cuschieri A 1979 Needle aspiration of the breast with immediate reporting of material. British Medical Journal 2: 185–187

Egan R L 1960 Experience with mammography in a tumour institute: evaluation of 1000 studies. Radiology 75: 894–900

Egan R L, Goldstein G T, McSweeney M M 1977 Conventional mammography, physical examination, thermography and xeroradiography in the detection of breast cancer. Cancer 39: 1984–1992

El-Domeiri A A, Shroff S 1976 Role of preoperative bone scan in carcinoma of the breast. Surgery, Gynecology and Obstetrics 142: 722–724

Feig S A 1984 Hypothetical breast cancer risk from mammography. In: Brunner S, Langfeldt B, Anderson P E (eds) Early detection of breast cancer. Springer-Verlag Berlin Heidelberg New York Tokyo Ch 1 p 1

Fisher B, Slack N, Katrych D 1975 Ten year follow-up results of patients with carcinoma of the breast in a co-operative clinical trial evaluating surgical adjuvant chemotherapy. Surgery, Gynecology and Obstetrics 140: 528–534

Fisher B 1977 Surgery of primary breast cancer. In: Maguire W L (ed) Breast cancer. Advances in research and treatment. Current approaches to therapy. Churchill Livingstone, Edinburgh London and New York Ch 1 p 1

Fisher B, Bauer M, Wickerham D, Redmond C, Fisher E 1983 Relation of number of positive axillary nodes to the prognosis of patients with primary breast cancer. An NSABP update. Cancer 52: 1551–1557

Franzen S, Zajicek J 1968 Aspiration biopsy in diagnosis of palpable lesions of the breast: critical review of 3479 consecutive biopsies. Acta Radiologica (Therapy) 7: 241–262

Galasko C S B 1975 The significance of occult skeletal metastases, detected by skeletal scintigraphy, in patients with otherwise apparently 'early' mammary carcinoma. British Journal of Surgery 62: 694–696

Gautherie M, Gros C M 1980 Breast thermography and cancer risk prediction. Cancer 45: 51–56

George W D, Burn J I 1975 Drill biopsy in the diagnosis of breast cancer. Clinical Oncology 1: 291–295

Hamilton T, Langlands A O, Prescott R J 1974 The treatment of operable cancer of the breast: a clinical trial in the South-east region of Scotland. British Journal of Surgery 61: 758–761

Harris J R, Levene M B, Hellman S 1978 The role of radiation therapy in the primary treatment of carcinoma of the breast. Seminars in Oncology 8: 408–416

Hughes L E, Webster D J T 1981 Reconstruction of the breast after mastectomy. Journal of the Royal Society of Medicine 74: 701–702

Isard H J, Becker W, Shilo R, Ostrum B J 1972 Breast thermography after 4 years and 10 000 studies. American Journal of Roentgenology 115: 811–821

Kaae S, Johansen H 1968 Simple versus radical mastectomy in primary breast cancer. In: Forrest A P M, Kunkler P B (eds) Prognostic factors in breast cancer, E and S Livingstone, Edinburgh. Part 2 p 93

Kline T S, Joshi L P, Neal H S 1979 Fine-needle aspiration of the breast: diagnosis and pitfalls. Cancer 44: 1458–1464

Landys K 1982 Prognostic value of bone marrow biopsy in breast cancer. Cancer 49: 513–518

Lapayowker M S, Revesz G 1980 Thermography and ultrasound in detection and diagnosis of breast cancer. Cancer 46: 933–938

Lee Y-T N 1981 Bone scanning in patients with early breast carcinoma: should it be a routine staging procedure? Cancer 47: 486–495

Leis H P 1980 Modified radical mastectomy: definition and role in breast cancer surgery. International Surgery 65: 211–218

Lewi H J, Roberts M M, Donaldson A A, Forrest A P M 1980 The use of cerebral computer assisted tomography as a staging investigation of patients with carcinoma of the breast and malignant melanoma. Surgery, Gynecology and Obstetrics 151: 385–386

Maddock W A, Carpenter J T, Laws H L 1982 Radical mastectomy versus modified radical mastectomy: a prospective, randomized trial in 311 breast cancer patients. Abstracts of the Twenty-eighth Annual Meeting of the Society of Surgical Oncology, Marco Island, 1982. p 60

Maguire G P, Lee E G, Bevington D J, Kuchemann C, Crabtree R J, Cornell C E 1978 Psychiatric problems in the first year after mastectomy. British Medical Journal 1: 963–965

Maguire P, Van Dam F 1983 Psychological aspects of breast cancery; workshop report. European Journal of Cancer and Clinical Oncology 19: 1735–1740

Mahoney L J, Bird B L, Cooke G M, Ball D G 1977 Early diagnosis of breast cancer: experience in a consultant breast clinic. Canadian Medical Association Journal 116: 1129–1131

Martin J E, Moskowitz M, Milbrath J R 1979 Breast cancer missed by mammography. American Journal of Roentgenology 132: 737–739

McNeil B J, Pace P D, Gray E B, Adelstein S J, Wilson R E 1978 Preoperative and follow-up bone scans in patients with primary carcinoma of the breast. Surgery, Gynecology and Obstetrics 147: 745–748

Meyerowitz B R, Roberts T, Volk H 1965 Pneumatic drill for tissue biopsy. American Journal of Surgery 109: 536–538

Meyerowitz B R 1976 Drill biopsy confirmation of breast cancer. Archives of Surgery 111: 826–827

Morris T 1983 Psychosocial aspects of breast cancer; a review. European Journal of Cancer and Clinical Oncology 19: 1725–1733

Moxley J H III, Allegra J C, Henney J, Muggia F 1980 Treatment of primary breast cancer. Journal of the American Medical Association 244: 797–800

Nash A G, Hurst P A E 1983 Central breast carcinoma treated by simultaneous mastectomy and latissimus dorsi flap reconstruction. British Journal of Surgery 70: 654–655

O'Connell M J, Wahner H W, Ahmann D L, Edis A J, Silvers A 1978 Value of preoperative radionuclide bone scan in suspected primary breast carcinoma. Mayo Clinic Proceedings 53: 221–226

Powell R W, McSweeney M B, Wilson C E 1983 X-ray calcifications as the only basis for breast biopsy. Annals of Surgery 197: 555–559

Preece P E, Baum M, Mansel R E, Webster D J T, Fortt R W, Gravelle I H et al 1982 Importance of mastalgia in operable breast cancer. British Medical Journal 284: 1299–1300

Rainsbury R M, Ott R J, Westwood J H, Coombes R C, Neville A M, Kalirai T S et al 1983 Location of metastatic breast carcinoma by a monoclonal antibody chelate labelled with indium-111. The Lancet: 1: 934–938

Redding W H, Coombes R C Monaghan P, Imrie S F, Ormerod M G, Gazet J, et al 1983 Detection of micrometastases in patients with primary breast cancer. The Lancet: 2: 1271–1273

Rimsten A, Stenkvist B, Joh anson H, Lindgren A 1975 The diagnostic accuracy of palpation and fine-needle biopsy and an evaluation of their combined use in the diagnosis of breast lesions. Annals of Surgery 182: 1–8

Roberts J G, Preece P E, Bolton P M, Baum M, Hughes L E 1975 The 'tru-cut' biopsy in breast cancer. Clinical Oncology 1: 297–303

Rosen P P, Fracchia A A, Urban J A, Schottenfeld D, Robbins G F 1975 'Residual' mammary carcinoma following simulated partial mastectomy. Cancer 35: 729–747

Shabot M M, Goldbery I M, Schick P, Nieberg R, Pilch Y H 1981 Aspiration cytology is superior to tru-cut needle biopsy establishing the diagnosis of clinically suspicious breast masses. Annals of Surgery 193: 122–126

Sickles E A, Klein D L, Goodson W H III, Hunt T K 1983a Mammography after needle aspiration of palpable breast masses. The American Journal of Surgery 145: 395–397

Sickles E A, Filly R A, Callen P W 1983b Breast cancer detection with sonography and mammography: comparison using state of the art equipment. American Journal of Roentgenology 140: 843–845

Simpson J S 1984 One-stage versus two-stage mastectomy, the patient's preference— Unpublished

Sterns E E, Curtis A C, Miller S, Hancock J R 1982 Thermography in breast diagnosis. Cancer 50: 323–325

Strawbridge H T G, Bassett A A, Foldes I 1981 Role of cytology in management of lesions of the breast. Surgery, Gynecology and Obstetrics 152: 1–7

Strax P, Venet L, Shapiro S 1973 Value of mammography in reduction of mortality for breast cancer in mass screening. American Journal of Roentgenology 117: 686–689

Tabar L, Dean P B, Péntek Z 1983 Galactography: the diagnostic procedure of choice for nipple discharge. Radiology 149: 31–38

Teixidor H S 1980 The use of ultrasonography in the management of masses of the breast. Surgery, Gynecology and Obstetrics 150: 486–490

Townsend C M Jr 1980 Breast lumps. Clinical Symposia 32: 3–33

Turner L, Swindell R, Bell W G T, Hartley R C, Tasker J H, Wilson W W et al 1981 Radical versus modified radical mastectomy for breast cancer. Annals of the Royal College of Surgeons England 63: 239–243

Veronesi U, Costa A 1982 The role of surgery in the management of primary breast cancer. In: Baum M (ed) Clinics in Oncology Volume 1 Number 3. Breast cancer. W B Saunders, London. Philadelphia Toronto Ch 9 p 853

Veronesi U, Valagussa P 1981 Inefficacy of internal mammary nodes dissection in breast cancer surgery. Cancer 47: 170–175

Veronesi U, Saccozzi R, Del Vecchio M, Banfi A, Clemente C, De Lena M, et al 1981 Comparing radical mastectomy with quadrantectomy, axillary dissection, and radiotherapy in patients with small cancers of the breast. New England Journal of Medicine 305: 6–11

Walker G M II, Foster R S, McKegney C P, McKegney F P 1978 Breast biopsy. A comparison of outpatient and inpatient experience. Archives of Surgery 113: 942–946

Watmough D J 1983 Transillumination of breast tissues: factors governing optimal imaging of lesions. Radiology 147: 89–92

Wiener S N, Sachs S H 1978 An assessment of routine liver scanning in patients with breast cancer. Archives of Surgery 113: 126–127

Yorkshire Breast Cancer Group 1983 Symptoms and signs of operable breast cancer 1976–1981. British Journal of Surgery 70: 350–351

12 Randomised trials of local treatment for breast cancer: overview and conclusions

R. J. C. STEELE

Introduction

Despite the prevailing and well-founded belief that breast cancer is a systemic disease by the time it is clinically detectable, there is little doubt that some form of local therapy is required. In a review of patients with untreated breast cancer, Bloom (1968) reported that 73% had marked ulceration of the breast at death, and that 21% had extensive destruction of the chest wall. He also pointed out that all untreated patients died from or with obvious tumour, and that their 5 year survival from onset of symptoms was 20%. These data can only lead us to conclude that the available local treatments for breast cancer can improve survival and morbidity, although nothing can be inferred about their effect on the incidence of metastatic disease. It still remains, however, to determine the optimum form of local therapy, and the most reliable information on which to base any conclusions comes from randomised, controlled clinical trials.

In this review, the local treatment options for breast cancer will be briefly described, and the results of randomised trials designed to evaluate surgical procedures and adjuvant radiotherapy will then be examined. Finally, a summary of the present position, with particular reference to the relationship between local and early systemic therapy will be presented.

Available methods of local treatment

Although evidence now exists that local removal of the tumour may be a rational surgical approach to breast cancer, mastectomy is still the standard treatment for this disease. As an adjunct to operation, the regional lymph node bearing areas may be excised, irradiated or left alone, and the skin flaps or residual breast tissue may also be treated by radiotherapy. Before embarking on an examination of the relative merits of the various approaches, it may be useful to define the terms which will be used.

157

Radical mastectomy
Although often attributed to Halstead (1898), this was first described by Moore in 1867. The breast, pectoralis major, pectoralis minor and the entire axillary contents are removed in the manner of a classical cancer operation.

Extended radical mastectomy
First described by Urban (1951), this procedure combines radical mastectomy with excision of the internal mammary node chain.

Modified radical mastectomy
Introduced by Patey and Dyson (1948), this operation involves removal of the breast and the axillary contents. Pectoralis major is left intact, but pectoralis minor may be removed or divided to facilitate access to the axilla (Scanlon & Caprini, 1975). The interpectoral (Rotter's) nodes may be left in this procedure, but a method of excising them through a fenestration in pectoralis major has been described (Croce, 1978).

Simple mastectomy
This involves removal of the entire breast without removal of the pectoral muscles. This operation may be supplemented by sampling the lower axillary lymph nodes (Forrest et al, 1976), but axillary clearance is avoided.

Tylectomy
This technique, often referred to as 'lumpectomy' simply involves local removal of the tumour with preservation of the breast. The procedure may be extended to a formal mammary quadrantectomy, but even then, cosmetically acceptable breast preservation may be achieved (Veronesi et al, 1981). Due to the multifocal nature of breast cancer, the risk of co-existent second primary tumours and the danger of leaving residual disease, however, it is generally agreed that tylectomy should be accompanied by radiotherapy.

Adjuvant radiotherapy
This is usually given as external beam megavoltage therapy to the axillary, supra- and infra-clavicular and parasternal node-bearing areas. It can be used as an adjuvant to simple mastectomy (McWhirter, 1948), or to radical mastectomy (Easson, 1968), and the usual dose is about 4500 cGy, although there is considerable variation in the literature. Radiotherapy given in conjunction with tylectomy may also be given as external beam radiotherapy (Veronesi et al, 1981), but implantation techniques using iridium wire can offer excellent local control (Prosnitz et al, 1977).

Chemotherapy
The role of chemotherapy lies with the treatment of systemic disease and cannot be regarded as a form of local control. Some workers have, however, attempted to ablate lymph node metastases using bleomycin emulsions, but this is still at an experimental stage (Tanigawa, 1980).

Randomised, controlled trials comparing surgical procedures

It is difficult to obtain information pertaining solely to the effect of surgical treatment on breast cancer, as most of the randomised trials comparing different surgical approaches are compounded by the application of radiotherapy. Nevertheless, it is possible to draw some conclusions from a few studies.

The Cardiff-St. Mary's trial (Forrest et al, 1977) compared simple mastectomy and node sampling to radical mastectomy in patients with histologically uninvolved nodes, and after follow-up for 3–9 years, no difference could be detected in survival rate or incidence of metastatic disease (Forrest et al, 1977). In this trial, patients with involved nodes were similarly randomised, but also received adjuvant radiotherapy, and again, no statistically significant difference was seen. This was not quite a fair comparison of surgical treatments, however, as the patients undergoing simple mastectomy had more limited radiotherapy. A similar difficulty is encountered with the Edinburgh trial (Langlands et al, 1980), where simple mastectomy with radiotherapy to the axillary, supraclavicular and parasternal regions was compared to radical mastectomy alone. The 12 year follow-up data demonstrated a significant prolongation of survival in the patients treated by the radical operation, but it is impossible to disentangle the relative effects of surgery and radiotherapy. This problem arises again in other studies where different surgical techniques were compared, but with radiotherapy as an adjunct to the more conservative approach (Kaae & Johansen, 1968; Fisher et al, 1978; Lythgoe & Palmer, 1982).

The Hammersmith trial is important in this context, as it compared simple mastectomy with radical mastectomy, both groups receiving similar radiotherapy to the axilla, clavicular and parasternal regions. The 5 year survival rates were 65% for the conservatively treated group and 70% for the radical group, but this difference was not statistically significant (Burn, 1974). Similarly, it is of interest to consider the report by Veronesi and Valagussa (1981), in which they give the results of a large multinational trial comparing radical mastectomy with extended radical mastectomy, no radiotherapy being used in either group. In this study, no differences in 5 or 10 year survival were noted.

While examining trials of surgical therapy in the local control of breast cancer, it is important to consider trials in which preservation of the breast has been an option. Several such studies are in progress, but the results of only two have been published. Firstly, the Guy's trial, comparing tylectomy with radical mastectomy in which both groups received post-operative radiotherapy, demonstrated no significant differences in either overall survival or distant recurrence at ten years (Hayward, 1977). This study is marred by a high local recurrence rate in the conservatively treated group, attributed to what would now be regarded as inadequate irradiation, but it is of interest that the incidence of generalised disease was not affected by removal of the axillary nodes. Unfortunately, it is not possible to determine the effect that metastatic involvement of the lymph nodes may have had on these two groups, as staging was carried out purely on clinical grounds. This problem may be overcome by combining local tumour excision with axillary dissection, and in the second available trial this has, in fact, been done. Between 1975 and 1980, 701 patients with tumours less than 2.0 cm in diameter were randomised to have a radical mastectomy or to undergo quadrantectomy with axillary dissection and 5000 cGy megavoltage external beam radiotherapy to the remaining breast tissue (Veronesi et al, 1981). Here, no differences in survival, disease-free survival or local recurrence were seen, and acceptable cosmetic results were reported in the conservatively treated group.

From the limited information available, it seems that surgical excision of loco-regional disease in breast cancer cannot alter the course of systemic dissemination. However, it is also important to examine its effect on local disease recurrence. Precise data are scanty, but Forrest (1977) reported that in patients with histologically negative nodes, those treated by simple mastectomy had a 13% axillary recurrence rate as opposed to a 4% rate in the radically-treated group; a difference almost certainly representing axillary metastases missed by the more conservative procedure. When radiotherapy was brought into the picture with the node-positive patients, the difference in local recurrence rates between the two types of operation was less, although in the Edinburgh trial (Langlands et al, 1980) radical mastectomy appeared to be superior to simple mastectomy in this respect. In the multinational trial (Veronesi & Valagussa, 1981), comparison of extended radical to radical mastectomy revealed that parasternal recurrence was only seen in the group treated by the lesser operation. However, this occurred in only 4% of cases, which was less than might be expected from the rate of internal mammary node involvement in patients treated by extended radical mastectomy.

It appears, then, that more extensive surgical procedures may spare a small proportion of patients the inconvenience of tumour recurrence in the regional nodes (Table 12.1). However, the advantage of radical surgery, even in this respect is not great, and it is therefore important to look at the question of morbidity.

Arm oedema and functional disability following radical mastectomy are well recognised (Watson et al, 1963; Burn, 1973), but comparisons must be made within randomised trials. Burn (1974) reported that the incidence of stiff shoulder and arm swelling was the same in patients treated by simple or radical mastectomy, but both groups were also given radiotherapy. On the other hand, analysis of arm elevation and arm diameter in patients treated within the Cardiff-St. Mary's trial showed a distinct advantage for simple mastectomy, both in irradiated and non-irradiated patients (Roberts et al, 1972). Such studies are sadly few, and more intensive investigation is required in this area.

Randomised, controlled trials designed to evaluate adjuvant radiotherapy

When examining the use of adjuvant radiotherapy in the local treatment of primary breast cancer, a major focus of interest is its effect on

Table 12.1 The effect of surgery on local lymph node recurrence in breast cancer.

Study	No. of patients with local recurrence in lymph nodes	P
Burn 1974		
Simple Mx and XRT	8/76	
Radical Mx and XRT	4/76	N.S.
Forrest et al 1977		
Simple Mx	10/75	
Radical Mx	3/79	N.S.
Simple Mx and XRT	2/49	
Radical Mx and XRT	2/40	N.S.
Langlands et al 1980		
Simple Mx and XRT	30/242	
Radical Mx	7/256	< 0.001
Veronesi & Valagussa 1981		
Radical Mx	15/374	
Extended radical Mx	0/342	< 0.001

Mx—Mastectomy
XRT—X-ray therapy

generalised recurrence and survival. There are many trials which have yielded important information in this respect, but, again, some are difficult to interpret owing to variation in the types of surgery and radiotherapy. Three trials have compared simple mastectomy and radiotherapy with radical or extended radical mastectomy alone. Two of these could demonstrate no difference in survival at 5 or at 10 years (Kaae & Johansen, 1968; Lythgoe & Palmer, 1982), but the Edinburgh trial (Langlands et al, 1980) produced a significant advantage for patients treated by radical mastectomy only, both in terms of absolute survival, and length of survival after the detection of metastases. In none of these studies is it possible to analyse the results according to pathological node status.

Fortunately, there are several randomised studies in which the surgical procedure was constant. Both the Manchester trial (Lythgoe & Palmer, 1982) and the King's/Cambridge trial (CRC Working Party, 1980) looked at the effect of radiotherapy with simple mastectomy, the former in clinical stage I patients only, and the latter in all operable cases. In neither study was there any difference in survival between the irradiated groups and the controls. Easson (1968) could demonstrate no difference in 10 year survival rates between patients given radiotherapy after radical mastectomy and those having surgery alone; histological node status had no effect on the distribution of these results. Similarly, Fisher and his colleagues (1970) found no advantage or disadvantage attached to adjuvant radiotherapy in the NSABP trial after 5 years of follow-up.

Wallgren, however, has reported promising results from the Stockholm trial which compared pre-operative radiotherapy, post-operative radiotherapy and no adjuvant treatment in patients undergoing modified radical mastectomy (Wallgren et al, 1980). In this study, the patients given pre-operative therapy had significantly improved survival over the controls, although those receiving post-operative irradiation were not advantaged. The Oslo trial, (Host & Brennhovd, 1977) which was designed to evaluate radiotherapy with radical mastectomy, has also produced some hopeful results. The first report suggested that distant metastases actually appeared earlier in node-positive patients when they were given radiotherapy. However, a later bulletin included the data of pertaining to cobalt-60 which produced a higher dose of radiation than the conventional X-ray technique used previously, and the cobalt-treated patients had a statistically significant survival advantage over the controls (Host & Brennhovd, 1977). Unfortunately, there are two flaws in this study. Firstly, the advantage was evident only at five years after treatment, and after this time the survival curves on the life table converged. Secondly, the controls used in the analysis included the controls from the earlier part of the trial when conventional X-rays were being used, so that the groups used for the comparison were not entirely contemporaneous.

The controversy over adjuvant radiotherapy has been prolonged, bitter, and, above all, unresolved (Montague & Fletcher, 1980; Lipsett, 1981). In a review of controlled trials, Stewart (1977) concluded that simple mastectomy and radiotherapy was as effective in terms of survival and recurrence rates as radical mastectomy with or without radiotherapy. In addition, she pointed out that post-operative radiotherapy did not prolong survival following radical mastectomy. However, the Edinburgh trial (Langlands et al, 1980) would now suggest that radical mastectomy may be slightly superior to simple mastectomy and radiotherapy, and to confuse matters further, the Stockholm and Oslo trials provide tentative evidence that radiotherapy may be a useful adjunct to radical or modified radical mastectomy (Deutsch, 1980).

Is it possible to resolve the dilemma by combining the available trial results? Such an approach has been used in the past by Stjernsward (1974), who brought together data from five trials, and, employing the Mantel-Haenzel procedure, showed a statistically significant decrease in 5 year survival for those receiving radiotherapy. This controversial publication was based on the combination of results from trials in which different forms of local surgery and radiotherapy had been used, and its validity was rightly criticised (Levitt et al, 1977). The concept of randomised controlled trials arose from the need to study contemporaneous populations, and to eliminate selection bias. Combining results from trials which are different in design and in temporal

Table 12.2 5 year survival figures in trials of adjuvant radiotherapy in which surgical treatment was not constant.

Trial	Therapy	5 year survival
Kaae & Johansen 1968	Extended radical Mx	138/206 (67%)
	Simple Mx and XRT	144/219 (66%)
Lythgoe & Palmer 1982 (Clinical Stage II)	Radical Mx	85/149 (57%)
	Simple Mx and XRT	87/159 (55%)
Langlands et al 1980	Radical Mx	192/256 (75%)
	Simple Mx and XRT	163/242 (67.5%)

Mx—Mastectomy
XRT—X-ray therapy

Table 12.3 5 year survival figures in trials of adjuvant radiotherapy in which a constant surgical procedure was used.

Trial	Therapy	5 year survival
Easson 1968	Radical Mx —no XRT —XRT	465/750 (62%) 410/707 (58%)
Fisher et al 1970	Radical Mx —no XRT —XRT	144/233 (62%) 109/195 (56%)
Host & Brennhovd 1977	Radical Mx —no XRT —XRT —Co-60	459/542 (85%) 231/281 (82%) 231/266 (87%)
CRC Working Party 1980	Simple Mx —no XRT —XRT	420/600 (70%) 434/594 (73%)
Wallgren et al 1980	Modified radical Mx —no XRT —XRT pre-op —XRT post-op	85/116 (73%) 91/116 (78%) 87/116 (75%)
Lythgoe & Palmer 1982 (Clinical Stage I)	Simple Mx —no XRT —XRT	248/359 (69%) 263/355 (74%)

Mx—Mastectomy
XRT—X-ray therapy

Table 12.4 Overall 5 year survival from combined trials of adjuvant radiotherapy.

Groups	5 year survival	
Groups with comparable surgical procedures only —no XRT —XRT	1821/2600 (70%) 1856/2630 (70%)	
By histological nodal status (all studies surgically comparable)	*Node −ve*	*Node +ve*
—no XRT	773/923 (84%)	342/600 (57%)
—XRT	701/869 (81%)	344/583 (59%)
Overall combination —no XRT —XRT	2236/3211 (70%) 2250/3250 (69%)	

XRT—X-ray therapy

and geographical situation, cannot, therefore, have any significance which is appropriate for statistical analysis. Nevertheless, it is important to examine the results of the available trials to determine whether there is an obvious collective trend. Tables 12.2 and 12.3 show the 5 year survival data from trials including adjuvant radiotherapy as an option, and Table 12.4 shows the combined results. No claims are made for the statistical validity of these data, but it is clear that no striking difference in 5 year survival exists between patients given adjuvant radiotherapy and those treated by surgery alone. It will be argued that statistically significant results have been seen in a few individual trials, but there is no doubt that the main body of evidence to date demonstrates that adjuvant radiotherapy has no major effect on the course of the disease in the general population suffering from breast cancer, irrespective of node status.

There is ample evidence, however, that radiotherapy consistently lowers the incidence of local recurrence after surgery (Easson, 1968; Fisher et al, 1970; Forrest et al, 1977; Host & Brennhovd, 1977; CRC Working Party, 1980; Wallgren et al, 1980; Lythgoe & Palmer, 1982). In some studies, 'local recurrence' is not further specified, but it is interesting to look at some trials in which nodal and chest wall recurrences were examined separately. Host and Brennhovd (1977) found that, after radical mastectomy, radiotherapy decreased the incidence of both chest wall and nodal recurrence in patients with involved nodes, although statistical significance existed only for nodal recurrence. Forrest and others (1977) noted that simple mastectomy with axillary radiotherapy was as effective as radical mastectomy and radical radiotherapy in controlling axillary node recurrence, but that the conservatively treated group had more chest wall recurrence. The Manchester study (Lythgoe & Palmer, 1982) has clearly shown that radiotherapy to the chest wall and regional nodes decreases both chest wall and axillary recurrence after simple mastectomy, but that simple mastectomy plus radiotherapy gives identical local control in both areas to radical mastectomy.

The case for radiotherapy as prophylaxis against local disease therefore seems strong, but the argument does not end here. Isolated local recurrence is quite rare, and its appearance usually heralds the onset of metastatic disease elsewhere (Dao & Nemoto, 1963; Bruce et al, 1970). This suggests that the appearance of local disease is purely a manifestation of actively enlarging systemic metastases, and, as such, it would not be expected to constitute a significant cause of death or morbidity in breast cancer, especially if it can be controlled by radiotherapy as it arises. Indeed, Easson (1968) has reported that delayed irradiation controlled local recurrence in a similar proportion of cases as did prophylactic radiotherapy, a finding endorsed by Stewart and her colleagues (1983) in a preliminary report of the second Edinburgh primary breast cancer trial. It is evident, therefore, that by withholding radiotherapy, the number of patients who will eventually require it can be reduced. Whether this is particularly desirable, however, depends on the morbidity attached to the procedure.

In the Cardiff-St. Mary's trial, it was found that patients receiving adjuvant radiotherapy were more likely to develop arm oedema and restriction of arm elevation in both the simple and radical mastectomy groups (Forrest et al, 1977). Similarly, Watson and his colleagues (1963) reported that, after radical mastectomy, arm swelling and impairment of function was commoner in irradiated patients. However, in both of these studies, only patients with involved axillary nodes were given radiotherapy, and it is not possible to differentiate between the effects of the two factors. De Schryver (1976), on the other hand, demonstrated an increased incidence of arm oedema and restriction of arm movement in all patients given pre- or post-operative radiotherapy compared to those treated by modified radical mastectomy alone within the Stockholm trial. Radiation to the chest wall can also lead to pulmonary complications (Oppedal & Kolbenstvedt, 1976) and it is also well known that the lymphangiosarcoma which can arise in lymphoedematous arms following radical mastectomy is usually seen where radiotherapy has also been given (Taswell et al, 1962).

Thus, there is no convincing evidence that treating the regional node bearing areas and the mastectomy skin flaps by radiotherapy confers any special benefit on breast cancer patients. Any argument for irradiation as prophylaxis against local recurrence after mastectomy can be countered by the extra morbidity suffered by many patients to no end.

Summary and conclusions

In summary, it appears that the degree of local therapy, in terms of either the extent of surgical excision or the addition of radiotherapy, has little effect on the course of breast cancer. This fits well with the concept of early systemic spread of the disease, and, of course, has contributed substantially towards it. Equally, there is no evidence that ablation of healthy lymph nodes draining breast cancer is detrimental, which seems to indicate that the effect of any local host reaction against the tumour in these nodes must be minimal. Obviously, however, local control of the tumour is important. When mastectomy is performed, there is still no evidence that giving radiotherapy at the time of operation is preferable to delaying the treatment until the first local recurrence; indeed, the latter course may be better, in view of the morbidity attached to irradiation. On the other hand, if tylectomy is to be a serious method of preserving mammary cosmesis, careful radiotherapy to the affected breast is vital in order to keep local recurrence rates at an acceptable level.

Clearly, breast conservation is now the direction in which the local therapy of early breast cancer is moving. Conceptually, there is every reason to expect that this will prove satisfactory, but the relevant randomised trials have still a long way to go before we have the definitive answer. In addition, before such conservative treatment can be accepted, these trials must provide evidence that the cosmetic results obtained are worth the effort.

In any appraisal of the local treatment of breast cancer, the systemic nature of the disease must not be overlooked. It is well known that adjuvant chemotherapy can improve disease-free survival rates (Fisher et al, 1975; Rossi et al, 1981), and recent trials of tamoxifen suggest that hormonal manipulation may provide an alternative and less toxic approach to early systemic therapy (Baum et al, 1983; Ribeiro & Palmer, 1983). In planning and analysing these trials it is important to have reliable prognostic information on the patients, and obtaining histological axillary node status is mandatory. The local treatment of breast cancer must therefore allow for this, and the relative merits of lower axillary sampling and total axillary clearance are still being debated. In a study by Davies and his colleagues (1980) post-operative examination of the lower nodes in total axillary clearance specimens failed to detect metastases in 14%

of cases which had tumour deposits in the higher nodes. Kissen and others (1982) performed 50 mastectomies with an axillary clearance preceded by lower axillary node sampling, and reported a 24% error rate in the sampling technique. This error, however, included patients in whom no nodes were identified. In contrast, a prospective, randomised trial of simple mastectomy and node sampling versus simple mastectomy and total axillary clearance is in progress in Edinburgh, and the results to date (Forrest et al, 1982) demonstrate that it is possible to identify nodes in every instance using a sampling technique, and that the incidence of node positivity is virtually identical in patients treated by sampling and clearance.

In concluding this review of randomised trials of local treatment for breast cancer, three main points can be made. Firstly, radical surgery is unnecessary. Secondly, radiotherapy reduces the rate of local recurrence after mastectomy, but delaying it until indicated by local recurrence is almost certainly safe and possibly preferable. Thirdly, breast conservation in early disease is a realistic option, but it has still to prove itself. It must be stressed, however, that the question of the ideal local therapy remains unresolved. New studies are in progress, and these will provide us with some of the answers, but we must not lose sight of the older trials—they have yet to reach maturity and they may well have surprises in store.

REFERENCES

Baum M et al 1983 Controlled trial of tamoxifen as adjuvant agent in management of early breast cancer. Lancet I: 257–261

Bloom H J G 1968 Survival of women with untreated breast cancer. In: Forrest A P M, Kunkler P B (eds) Prognostic Factors in Breast Cancer. E & S Livingstone, Edinburgh & London. p 3–19

Bruce J, Carter D C, Fraser J 1970 Patterns of recurrent disease in breast cancer. Lancet I: 433–435

Burn J I 1973 Mechanical effects of lymphadenectomy. Journal of the Royal College of Surgeons of Edinburgh 18: 346–350

Burn J I 1974 'Early' breast cancer: the Hammersmith trial. British Journal of Surgery 61: 762–765

CRC Working Party 1980 Cancer Research Campaign (King's/Cambridge) trial for early breast cancer. Lancet II: 55–60

Croce E J 1978 A neoclassical radical mastectomy. Surgery, Gynecology and Obstetrics 147: 921–923

Dao T L, Nemoto T 1963 The clinical significance of skin recurrence after radical mastectomy in women with cancer of the breast. Surgery, Gyneocology and Obstetrics 117: 447–453

Davies G C, Millis R R, Hayward J L 1980 Assessment of axillary lymph node status. Annals of Surgery 192: 148–151

De Schryver A 1976 The Stockholm breast cancer trial: preliminary report of a randomised study concerning the value of pre-operative or postoperative radiotherapy in operable disease. International Journal of Radiation Oncology, Biology, Physics 1: 601–609

Deutsch M 1980 Breast cancer: adjuvant radiotherapy revisited. International Journal of Radiation Oncology, Biology, Physics 6: 389–391

Easson E C 1968 Post-operative radiotherapy in breast cancer. In: Forrest A P M, Kunkler P B (eds) Prognostic Factors in Breast Cancer. E & S Livingstone, Edinburgh & London. p 118–127

Fisher B, Slack N H, Cavanagh P J, Gardener B, Ravdin R G 1970 Postoperative radiotherapy in the treatment of breast cancer: results of the NSABP clinical trial. Annals of Surgery 172: 711–732

Fisher B et al 1975 L-PAM in the management of primary breast cancer: a report of the early findings. New England Journal of Medicine 292: 117–122

Fisher B, Redmond C, Fisher E R 1978 Clinical trials and the surgical treatment of breast cancer. Surgical Clinics of North America 58: 723–736

Forrest A P M, Roberts M M, Cant E, Shivas A A 1976 Simple mastectomy and pectoral node biopsy. British Journal of Surgery 63: 569–575

Forrest A P M et al 1977 Simple mastectomy and pectoral node biopsy: the Cardiff-St. Mary's trial. World Journal of Surgery 1: 320–323

Forrest A P M, Steele R J C, Stewart H J 1982 Axillary sampling in breast cancer. Lancet II: 38

Halstead W 1898 A clinical and histological study of certain adenocarcinomata of the breast. Transactions of the Americal Surgical Association 16: 144–181

Hayward J L 1977 The Guy's trial of treatments of 'early' breast cancer. World Journal of Surgery 1: 314–316

Host H, Brennhovd I O 1977 The effect of postoperative radiotherapy in breast cancer. International Journal of Radiation Oncology, Biology, Physics 2: 1061–1067

Kaae S, Johansen H 1968 Simple versus radical mastectomy in primary breast cancer. In: Forrest A P M, Kunkler P B (eds) Prognostic Factors in Breast Cancer. E & S Livingstone, Edinburgh & London. p 93–102

Kissen M W, Thompson E M, Price A B, Slavin G, Kark A E 1982 The inadequacy of axillary sampling in breast cancer. Lancet I: 1210–1212

Langlands A G, Prescott R J, Hamilton T 1980 A clinical trial in the management of operable cancer of the breast. British Journal of Surgery 67: 170–174

Levitt S H, McHugh R B, Song C W 1977 Radiotherapy in the post-operative treatment of operable cancer of the breast. Cancer 39: 924–940

Lipsett M B 1981 Post-operative radiation for women with cancer of the breast and positive lymph nodes: should it continue? New England Journal of Medicine 304: 112–114

Lythgoe J P, Palmer M K 1982 Manchester regional breast study—5 and 10 year results. British Journal of Surgery 69: 693–696

McWhirter R 1948 The value of simple mastectomy and radiotherapy in the treatment of cancer of the breast. British Journal of Radiology 21: 599–610

Montague E, Fletcher G H 1980 The curative value of irradiation in the treatment of nondisseminated breast cancer. Cancer 46: 995–998

Moore C H 1867 On the influence of inadequate operations on the theory of breast cancer. Proceedings of the Royal Medico-Chirurgical Society of London 1: 245–250

Oppedal T, Kolbenstvedt A 1976 Pulmonary contraction following ^{60}Co irradiation of mammary carcinoma. Acta Radiologica (Therapy, Physics, Biology) 15: 329–336

Patey D H, Dyson W H 1948 The prognosis of carcinoma of the breast in relation to the type of operation performed. British Journal of Cancer 2: 7–13

Prosnitz L R et al 1977 Radiation therapy as initial treatment for early stage cancer of the breast without mastectomy. Cancer 39: 917–923

Ribeiro G, Palmer M K 1983 Adjuvant tamoxifen for operable carcinoma of the breast: report of clinical trial by the Christie Hospital and Holt Radium Institute. British Medical Journal 286: 827–830

Roberts M M, Furnival I G, Forrest A P M 1972 The morbidity of mastectomy. British Journal of Surgery 59: 301–302

Rossi A, Bonadonna G, Valagussa P, Veronesi U 1981 Multimodal treatment in operable breast cancer: five year results of the CMF program. British Medical Journal 282: 1427–1431

Scanlon E F, Caprini J A 1975 Modified radical mastectomy. Cancer 35: 710–713

Stewart H J 1977 Controlled trials in the treatment of 'early' breast cancer: a review of the published results. World Journal of Surgery 1: 309–313

Stewart H J et al 1983 Mastectomy and node sampling: the need for postoperative radiotherapy. British Journal of Surgery 70: 692

Stjernsward J 1974 Decreased survival related to irradiation post-operatively in early operable breast cancer. Lancet II: 1285–1286

Tanigawan N et al 1980 Surgical chemotherapy against lymph node metastases: an experimental study. Surgery 87: 147–152

Taswell H F, Soule E H, Coventry M B 1962 Lymphangiosarcoma arising in chronic lymphoedematous extremities. Journal of Bone and Joint Surgery 44A: 277–294

Urban J A 1951 Radical excision of the chest wall for breast cancer. Cancer 4: 1263–1285

Veronesi U, Valagussa P 1981 Inefficacy of internal mammary node dissection in breast cancer surgery. Cancer 47: 170–175

Veronesi U et al 1981 Comparing radical mastectomy with quadrantectomy, axillary dissection and radiotherapy in patients with small cancers of the breasts. New England Journal of Medicine 305: 6–11

Wallgren A et al 1980 The value of pre-operative radiotherapy in operable mammary carcinoma. International Journal of Radiation Oncology, Biology, Physics 6: 287–290

Watson T A, Bond A F, Phillips A J 1963 Swelling and dysfunction of the upper limb following radical mastectomy. Surgery, Gynecology and Obstetrics 116: 99–104

13 *Locally advanced disease: integrated management*

ALLAN O. LANGLANDS

It is conventional to define four stages of breast cancer of differing prognosis by criteria applied to the primary tumour, the regional lymph nodes and the presence or absence of distant metastases. However, for the clinician concerned with the development of primary treatment strategies, it is useful to consider only three categories of disease which pose fundamental therapeutic questions (Table 13.1). It is clear from a consideration of Table 13.1 that the conventional stages of the disease do not define these clinical categories at all precisely and that the therapeutic objectives, and thus the requirements for the evaluation of treatment outcome, are very different in each.

Table 13.1 A comparison between the clinical categories of breast cancer, the appropriate therapeutic objective for each and current problems in defining management strategies.

Extent of disease	Category	Therapeutic objective	Current problems
$T_{1-3} N_0 M_0$	'Operable' or 'Early'	Cure	Extent of primary treatment required. Management of sub-clinical micrometastatic disease
$T_{3-4} N_{0-3} M_0$	'Locally advanced' or 'Inoperable'	Local disease control	Definition of the category. Integration of treatment modalities.
$T_{any} N_{any} M_1$	Metastatic	Symptom control	Overtreatment, particularly by chemotherapy.

It is also clear from Table 13.1 that any consideration of the management of locally advanced breast cancer must deal in detail with three aspects, namely the categorisation of this clinical entity and its natural history, its management, and the definition of the most appropriate measures of treatment outcome. All of these are major sources of confusion in the literature on breast cancer, either because of their intrinsic imprecision or because of variability in their clinical application (Table 13.2).

Table 13.2 Sources of confusion in the literature regarding the definition of locally advanced breast cancer and it treatment.

Definition of the Category	TNM Surgical opinion. Inclusion or exclusion of inflammatory carcinoma.
Treatment	Toilet mastectomy. Highly variable radiation therapy (technique and dose). Endocrine therapy. Highly variable chemotherapy. Inclusion in protocols for metastatic or recurrent disease.
Outcome	Control of local disease. Quality of life. Survival.

Definition of the category

It is illogical and unscientific to attempt to define this category of breast cancer in terms of a single treatment modality, ie as 'inoperable disease' and the term locally advanced disease is preferable. The criteria of operability vary widely from 50.6% of cases deemed 'unsuitable for surgery' after triple node biopsy (Guttman, 1967) through 80% of cases capable of treatment by simple mastectomy, usually with post-operative radiation (Langlands et al, 1976) to around 90% of cases referred to an institution where standard treatment would be by radical mastectomy (Chu, 1974).

It is equally illogical to attempt to define this category in terms of the primary tumour alone and some account must be taken in the development of treatment strategies of patients who present with early ('operable') disease but in whom extensive involvement of the axillary nodes is found in the operative specimen. The probabilities for the control of local disease and for survival deteriorate steadily as the number of nodes involved increases (Nemoto et al, 1980; Rao et al, 1982) and current practice to sub-divide cases, from the point of view of prognosis, into those with three or less, and those with more than three involved nodes, merely represents clinical convenience as no true watershed exists. A problem remains in the inclusion of the extent of lymph node involvement in the definition of locally advanced disease. This obviously includes cases with fixed axillary nodes, and/or supraclavicular nodes, but should also include those patients with large numbers of nodes, say more than 10, found to be positive in an operative specimen.

Although the TNM configuration is useful, it does not permit precise definition of this category of the disease. As a generalisation however, locally advanced breast cancer includes categories covered by T_3N_{2-3}, T_4N_{0-3}, M_0.

The natural history of locally advanced disease

Estimates of the frequency with which locally advanced disease is found differ as a result of variability in the definition of the category. Langlands et al (1976) so classified 8.5% of 1941 cases of breast cancer seen in a 5 year period and Rubens et al (1977), 17% of all cases seen in a 13 year period but Carbone and Davis (1978) have suggested that the proportion of patients with locally advanced or inflammatory carcinoma at presentation may be as high as 15–25%. However since breast cancer itself is common, patients with locally advanced disease pose a numerically greater problem in a department of radiation oncology than, for example, do patients with cancer of the thyroid, testicular tumours or Hodgkin's disease. This fact alone makes the separate, detailed consideration of their management worthwhile.

The imprecisions in the definition of this form of breast cancer are reflected in considerable variation in the reporting of its natural history. 5 year survival rates varying from 1% (Nohrman, 1949) to over 20% (Rubens, 1978) have been recorded in series treated mainly by radiotherapy. When primary radiation therapy is followed by mastectomy in selected cases the survival rate rises to around 30% (Zucali et al, 1976).

The median survival of 25–30 months of patients with disease classified at $T_{3-4} N_X M_0$, treated mainly by radiation therapy (Zucali et al, 1976; Rubens et al, 1977), is not significantly different from that of 2.7 years for patients with *operable* $T_3 N_{0-1} M_0$ disease (Langlands & Kerr, 1978) nor indeed does it differ from the median survival of patients with untreated breast cancer in the late 19th and early 20th centuries (Bloom et al, 1968). This suggests that the controversy which exists regarding the results of the treatment of locally advanced disease by radiotherapy, alone or in combination with surgery, is specious and that survival is unaffected by the form of local therapy. If this is so, it follows that the criterion by which therapy should be evaluated is its ability to control the local manifestations of the disease.

There is not a great deal of information on the prognostic significance of menstrual status. It did not significantly affect outcome in two studies of multimodality therapy (De Lena et al, 1981; Hortobagyi et al, 1983) in spite of the latter study including patients in 80% of whom tumours were oestrogen receptor positive. On the other hand, all 5 year survivors among 165 cases treated by X-ray therapy were at least 5 years post-menopausal (Langlands et al, 1980) and Rubens et al (1977) reported a reduced survival in women within 5 years of the menopause. Buzdar et al (1981) failed to show an improvement in the survival of patients aged less than 50 with inflammatory carcinoma, treated by a combined modality approach, largely due to the high incidence of central nervous system relapse in younger patients.

It is also difficult to analyse the significance of different clinical features which, either alone or in combination, place a patient in the locally advanced category. A large ($\geq$ 8 cm) primary tumour, involvement of supraclavicular lymph nodes, the presence of extensive skin involvement by oedema (peau d'orange), satellite nodules in the skin of the breast and the subcategory of inflammatory breast cancer are all associated with a further reduction in survival expectation and, until the advent of chemotherapy, with poor prospects for the local control of disease (Langlands & Kerr, 1978; Rao et al, 1982).

The diagnosis of inflammatory carcinoma of the breast is usually made on clinical grounds with enlargement of the breast, pain, redness and oedema of the skin, though some would argue that a sine qua non is the histological demonstration of tumour in dermal lymphatics (Ellis & Teitelbaum, 1974). Inflammatory carcinoma of the breast, however defined, is rare accounting perhaps for 1–2% of all cases of breast cancer (Stocks & Patterson, 1976). As a corollary experience in its management must be gathered over many years during which the assessment of disease and its treatment could vary considerably. Depending on the criteria accepted for its definition and to a lesser extent on treatment, the 5 year survival rates reported range from 0–14%.

When radiation therapy was the standard treatment results were so poor that the management of inflammatory carcinoma was conventionally considered separately. The current recommendation (1982) in the TNM staging system is that this convention is continued. However, with the introduction of chemotherapy into treatment strategies for the management of locally advanced disease, the exclusion from the study of patients with inflammatory carcinoma has become less common and has thus further complicated the comparisons of treatment outcome.

Treatment

Radiotherapy

Until relatively recently radiotherapy was the mainstay of treatment for patients with locally advanced disease. Breast cancer is a moderately radiosensitive tumour and even bulky disease is capable of control by radiation therapy for considerable periods of time (Chu, 1974; Langlands et al, 1976; Strickland, 1973; Zucali et al, 1976).

The ability to control local disease by X-ray therapy led to the comparison of the results of radiation treatment with those from the surgical management of a dissimilar group of cases. This has meant an over-concentration on survival data and a tendency to ignore important issues such as the duration of local control of a disease, the treatment of which is palliative. The position is further complicated by considerable variation in cases selected for radiation therapy and its erratic use as a pre-operative measure. Consistently improved survival in those patients undergoing mastectomy subsequently (Caldwell, 1971; De Larue et al, 1965; Rao et al, 1982; Zucali et al, 1976) obviously reflects case selection but it has promoted the inclusion of cases with a relatively good prognosis in 'inoperable' series and has sustained unprofitable debate regarding combined therapy.

In a review of eight series, totalling 1822 cases, treated by radiation therapy, variably combined with surgery but with no case receiving chemotherapy, the mean 5 year survival was 21.5% (Rubens, 1978). Since a significant proportion of patients survies for more than 3 years the duration of local control is an important factor determining the quality of a patient's life. Good palliation, as measured by the control of ulceration, bleeding or discharge was achieved from a dose of 30 Gy in 5 fractions in 2 weeks (NSD 1500–1560) but only 19% of patients so treated had control of local disease at death. When the dose was increased to 45 Gy in 10 fractions in 4 weeks (NSD 1724–1796) local disease was controlled at death in 41% of cases (Langlands et al, 1976). Higher local control rates may be obtained in selected patients suitable for further increased dosage from interstitial implant (Bruckman et al, 1979) though Spanos et al

(1980) found unacceptably high complication rates (severe fibrosis and/or necrosis) when high doses were used to give a loco-regional control rate of 72%.

Two studies, in which twice daily treatment was used in the management of inflammatory carcinoma, have reported a significant reduction in loco-regional failure, from 46% to 27% (Barker et al, 1980) and from 69% to 33% (Chu et al, 1980) compared to conventional, once-daily fractionation.

These figures are a convincing argument for the use of radical radiation therapy schedules whenever possible and the use of lower doses should be restricted to the short-term palliation of the frail or elderly patient. Similarly they are an argument against rapid high dose techniques (20–25 Gy in two or three fractions) (Atkins, 1964; Edelman et al, 1965; Stoll, 1965). This approach is associated with a considerably increased morbidity from fibrosis of the breast, lymphoedema and/or damage to the underlying lung.

Surgery

In 1943 Haagensen and Stout published a retrospective analysis of the results of radical surgery in 120 cases of locally advanced disease. The 5 year survival rate was 1% and the local recurrence rate 49.2%. Their criteria of inoperability defined from that time a subset of patients in whose treatment surgery appeared to have no primary role (Stoker, 1974). These patients were traditionally treated by radiation therapy and more recently by chemotherapy. Both can produce impressive local control of disease and as a result both have been used as adjuncts to surgery. However, it is clear that two factors combine to give an apparent improvement in survival in cases treated by surgery. Firstly, there is selection for this approach of patients who have less extensive disease and secondly, there is selection of patients for surgery who exhibit good tumour control by the other modality. To date there is no convincing evidence that the consistently higher survival rates reported for cases treated by mastectomy following a response to radiation or chemotherapy are due to other than case-selection. The studies reported by De Lena et al (1978, 1981) showed that chemotherapy (4 cycles of adriamycin and vincristine) yielded a response rate of around 90%. When those cases showing a response to chemotherapy then underwent radical radiation therapy, 81% (or 73% of all patients entering the study) achieved complete remission of disease. When cases showing a response to chemotherapy were randomised to subsequent surgery or radiation therapy no advantage was demonstrated for those undergoing mastectomy either in local control of disease or survival. It is doubtful therefore whether radical surgery has a major role in the management of locally advanced disease either as a definitive procedure with or without radiation therapy or chemotherapy, or as the so called toilet mastectomy to remove, as a palliative measure, fungating or discharging tumour. There is a real risk of uncontrolled local disease resulting from injudicious surgery.

Chemotherapy

Breast cancer is a moderately chemosensitive tumour. Once this was established in studies on patients with metastatic disease, it was logical to introduce chemotherapy into the management of locally advanced disease, almost always in combination with radiation therapy. Important conclusions can be drawn regarding the role of chemotherapy in a combined modality approach to locally advanced disease (De Lena et al, 1981; Rubens et al, 1980; Serrou et al, 1979).

1. When combination chemotherapy (3–4 cycles) is followed by radical radiation therapy over 80% of those showing a response to chemotherapy achieve a complete remission of local disease which may be maintained for considerable periods of time.

2. The duration of this disease-free survival is significantly increased over cases treated by radiation therapy alone.

3. There is no advantage from carrying out radical surgery as opposed to radical radiotherapy following initial chemotherapy.

4. Radiation therapy and chemotherapy can successfully be combined in treatment protocols with acceptable toxicity.

5. There is an advantage, in terms of disease control, in further chemotherapy following the induction of a complete remission.

Claims that improved control of local disease occurs when radiation therapy follows initial treatment by multi-agent chemotherapy delivered via a subclavian artery catheter (Stephens et al, 1980) are not supported by data on a sufficient number of patients. Furthermore a pharmacodynamic rationale for the superiority of this more complex approach remains to be established (Chen & Gross, 1980).

Table 13.3 shows four chemotherapy regimes in common use in the management of advanced breast cancer, the response rates being derived from clinical trial data. Regimes based on adriamycin on average have a higher response rate to those based on cyclophosphamide but other (disturbing) comparisons can be made. The range of response rates is considerable and a statistically significant difference exists, for three of the four regimes, when the lowest and highest response rates are compared. This is probably due to the small number of cases in the average trial (46) and, more importantly, to the heterogeneity of cases selected for treatment and the imprecision inherent in its assessment.

Table 13.3 The response rates derived from clinical trials of four regimes in common use in advanced breast cancer. A statistically significant difference exists between the lowest and highest response rates for three of the four regimes. For CMFVP the lowest and highest response rates were recorded in different trials by the same investigator.

Regime	No. of trials	No. of cases	Response rate % (Range)
AC	3	55	53 (44–60)[a]
AV	3	110	46 (25–67)[b]
CMF	4	197	43 (24–63)[c]
CMFVP	6	380	48 (32*–64*)[c]

*Different trials by same investigator
a = Not significant
b = P<0.05
c = P<0.01

When account is taken of the fact that patients with locally advanced disease present with an excessive tumour burden, these findings are cogent reasons why trials in the management of locally advanced disease which seek to compare the impact of relatively minor variations in chemotherapy regimes of broadly comparable efficiency are unlikely to produce significant results (Bonadonna & Valagussa, 1983). Differences which inevitably emerge would be more likely than not to represent the play of chance magnified by the considerable variability in the behaviour of this category of breast cancer. Nevertheless several clinical trials have been established and these are tabulated in summary form in Table 13.4.

Hormone therapy

The recent advances made in the treatment of breast cancer by chemotherapy have tended to overshadow important developments in hormone therapy. This is perhaps unreasonable since, irrespective of the aggressiveness of any approach to the management of locally advanced disease, it must always be remembered that treatment can only be palliative. Tamoxifen has proved to be an effective agent in the management of advanced and recurrent breast cancer particularly in oestrogen receptor positive cases. Its conspicuous lack of toxicity makes it an attractive 'soft option' which may be employed initially, particularly in elderly or frail patients (Preece et al, 1982). Furthermore aminoglutethamide is predictably an effective treatment in a large proportion

Table 13.4 Six current clinical trials in the management of locally advanced breast cancer (modified from Compilation of Experimental Cancer Therapy Protocol Summaries, 1983). The basic structure of chemotherapy-radiotherapy-chemotherapy is unlikely to yield any significant difference in survival which is dependent on the chemotherapy under study.

CLB 7784

```
                    RM
   CAFVP × 3 →      vs    → CAFVP → CMFVP for 2 years
                    XRT
```

EST 3181

```
                         XRT
   RM → CAFTH × 6 →      vs
                         OBSERVATION − XRT on relapse
```

EST 8177

```
   CMFP × 3 + XRT
         vs              → responders CMFP × 18
       XRT
```

MDAR 259—MDA 7807

```
   Escalating FAC (protected environment + antibiotics)
         vs                                              −CMF × 24
   Standard FAC
```

EORTC 10792

```
                    Hormone Therapy
                    CMFP × 8
   RT → Responders →
                    CMFP + Hormone therapy
                    Observation
```

PERU-INEN 7804

```
                                        CMF + Lev
   CMF + XRT + CMF × 6                       vs        × 12
         vs                                 CMF
   RM + CMF × 6 + XRT
```

of patients who relapse after a response to Tamoxifen, and is relatively non-toxic compared to chemotherapy.

The more aggressive combined modality approach could then be reserved for younger, fitter patients, those with inflammatory carcinoma, those known to be receptor negative or those who fail to respond to the simpler hormonal manipulation. See Figure 13.1.

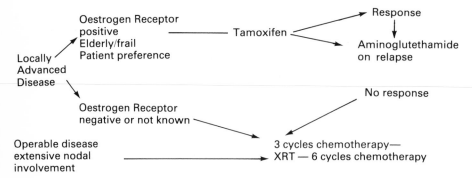

Fig. 13.1 A scheme for the management of locally extensive (defined according to the number of nodes involved) or locally advanced breast cancer. The scheme accepts that locally advanced disease is incurable and that disease control is the main therapeutic objective.

Immunotherapy

The fact that locally advanced breast cancer represents (by definition) bulky local disease in the absence of systemic spread may be taken to indicate disease of a different biological potential. This, and the fact that normal T-lymphocyte counts are found in patients with Stage III disease in contrast to depressed levels in all other patients, including those with the earliest tumours, have suggested the operation of immunological factors (Whitehead et al, 1976) and have prompted attempts to include immunotherapy in a combined modality approach.

BCG (Hortobagyi et al, 1983; Perloff & Lesnick, 1982) levamisole (Olivari et al, 1980) and intravenous C parvum (Chare et al, 1977) have been evaluated with conflicting results. The most impressive claim for significantly improved survival comes from Olivari et al. However this must be accepted with caution in view of the report by Brincker et al (1980) of an increased recurrence rate in patients with operable disease who received levamisole after mastectomy and radiotherapy, compared to those who did not.

As a generalisation, immunotherapy as a single treatment is associated with negligible response rates and significant toxicity (Chare et al, 1977; Serrou et al, 1979) and its use is usually as part of a complex protocol including chemotherapy and/or radiotherapy. In that reported by Hortobagyi et al (1983) only 14 out of 52 patients completed treatment so that no valid conclusion can be drawn regarding the contribution of the immunotherapy component. However a 60 per cent failure at 5 years suggest that this complex and toxic protocol has no advantage over simpler approaches.

Since this chapter was written, the 5-year results of the NSABP trial comparing total mastectomy with segmental mastectomy have been published (Fisher et al, 1985). In this trial, 1843 patients with tumours of 4 cm or less were randomised to have a total mastectomy, a segmental mastectomy or a segmental mastectomy with radiotherapy, and all node positive patients were given adjuvant chemotherapy. No differences were observed between the three groups in overall survival without distant metastases. This study clearly indicates that local tumour excision with adequate radiotherapy can provide acceptable disease control, at least in the first 5 years. If prolonged follow-up reveals continuation of these trends, and if the cosmetic result is conclusively shown to be an improvement on mastectomy, then local tumour excision supplemented by irradiation may be regarded as the optimum available treatment for small breast cancers.

REFERENCES

Atkins H L 1964 Massive dose technique in radiation therapy of inoperable carcinoma of the breast. American Journal of Roentgenology 91: 80–89

Barker J L, Montague E D, Peters L J 1980 Clinical experience with irradiation of inflammatory carcinoma of the breast with and without elective chemotherapy. Cancer 45: 625–629

Bloom H J G 1968 Survival of women with breast cancer—past and present. In: Forrest A P M, Kunkler P B (eds) Prognostic factors in breast cancer. E & S Livingstone, Edinburgh p 3–19

Bonadonna G, Valagussa P 1983 Chemotherapy of breast cancer: current views and results. International Journal of Radiation Oncology Biology and Physics 9: 279–297

Brincker H, Mouridsen H T, Andersen K W 1980 Increased breast cancer recurrence rate after adjuvant therapy with levamisole. The Lancet II: 824–827

Bruckman J E, Harris J R, Levene M B, Chaffey J T, Hellman S 1979 Results of treating Stage III carcinoma of the breast by primary radiation therapy. Cancer 43: 985–993

Buzdar A U, Montague E D, Barker J L, Hortobagyi G N, Blumenschein G R 1981 Management of inflammatory carcinoma of breast with combined modality approach—an update. Cancer 47: 2537–2542

Caldwell W L 1971 Preoperative irradiation for locally advanced breast cancer. Cancer 28: 1647–1650

Carbone P P, Davis R E 1978 Medical treatment for advanced breast cancer. Seminars in Oncology 4: 417–427

Chare M J B, Webster D J T, Baum M 1977 Clinical experience in the use of C parvum in the treatment of locally advanced carcinoma of the breast. Developments in Biological Standardization 38: 495–499

Chen H-S, Gross J F 1980 Intra-arterial infusion of anti-cancer drugs: theoretic aspect of drug delivery and review of responses. Cancer Treatment Reports 64: 31–40

Chu F C H 1974 Current policies of radiation therapy of breast cancer. Clinical Bulletin 4: 108–111

Chu A M, Wood W D, Doucette J A 1980 Inflammatory breast carcinoma treated by radical radiotherapy. Cancer 45: 2730–2737

Compilation of Experimental Cancer Therapy Protocol Summaries 1983. U S Department of Health and Human Services, National Institutes of Health

De Larue N C, Ash C L, Peters V, Fielden R 1965 Pre-operative radiation in the management of locally advanced breast cancer. Archives of Surgery 91: 136–154

De Lena M, Varini M, Zucali R et al 1981 Multimodal treatment for locally advanced breast cancer. Results of chemotherapy-radiotherapy versus chemotherapy-surgery. Cancer Clinical Trials 4: 229–236

De Lena M, Zucali R, Viganotti G, Valagussa P, Bonadonna G 1978 Combined chemotherapy-radiotherapy in locally advanced (T_{3b}–T_4) breast cancer. Cancer Chemotherapy and Pharmacology 1: 53–59

Edelman A J, Holtz S, Powers W E 1965 Rapid radiotherapy for inoperable carcinoma of the breast. American Journal of Roentgenology 93: 585–599

Ellis D L, Teitelbaum S L 1974 Inflammatory carcinoma of the breast: a pathologic definition. Cancer 33: 1045–1047

Fisher B et al 1985 Five year results of a randomised trial comparing total mastectomy and segmental mastectomy with or without radiation in the treatment of breast cancer. New England Journal of Medicine 312: 665–673

Guttman R 1967 Radiotherapy in locally advanced cancer of the breast. Adjunct to standard therapy. Cancer 20: 1046–1050

Haagensen C D, Stout A P 1943 Carcinoma of the breast II. Criteria of operability. Annals of Surgery 118: 859–870

Hortobagyi G N, Blumenschein G R, Spanos W et al 1983 Multimodal treatment of locoregionally advanced breast cancer. Cancer 51: 763–768

Langlands A O, Forbes J F, Tattersall M H N 1980 The treatment of locally advanced breast cancer; a discussion document. Australasian Radiology 24: 307–310

Langlands A O, Kerr G R 1978 Prognosis in breast cancer: the relevance of clinical staging. Clinical Radiology 29: 599–606

Langlands A O, Kerr G R, Shaw S 1976 The management of locally advanced breast cancer by X-ray therapy. Clinical Oncology 2: 365–371

Nemoto T, Vana J, Bedwani R N et al 1980 Management and survival of female breast cancer. Cancer 45: 2917–2924

Nohrman B A 1949 Cancer of the breast. A clinical study of 1042 cases treated at Radiumhemmit, 1936–41. Acta Radiologica Supplement 77: 62–63

Olivari A J, Glait H M, Varela O A, Feierstein J N 1980 Six years follow-up in levamisole treated Stage III breast cancer patients. Proceedings of the American Association for Clinical Oncology C172

Perloff M, Lesnick G J 1982 Chemotherapy before and after mastectomy in Stage III breast cancer. Archives of Surgery 117: 879–881

Preece P E, Wood R A B, Mackie C R, Cuschieri A 1982 Tamoxifen as initial sole treatment for localised breast cancer in elderly women: a pilot study. British Medical Journal 284: 869–870

Rao D V, Bedwinek J, Perez C, Lee J, Fineberg B 1982 Prognostic indicators in Stage III and localised Stage IV breast cancer. Cancer 50: 2037–2043

Rubens R D 1978 Systemic therapy combined with radiotherapy for primary inoperable carcinoma of the breast. Applications of Cancer Chemotherapy 24: 205–212

Rubens R D, Armitage P, Winter P J, Tong D, Hayward J L 1977 Prognosis in inoperable Stage III carcinoma of the breast. European Journal of Cancer 13: 805–811

Rubens R D, Sexton S, Tong D, Winter P J, Knight R K, Hayward J L 1980 Combined chemotherapy and radiotherapy for locally advanced breast cancer. European Journal of Cancer 16: 351–356

Serrou B, Sancho-Garnier H, Cappalaere P 1979 Results of a randomised trial of prophylactic chemotherapy in T_3–T_4 breast cancer patients previously treated by radiotherapy. Recent Results in Cancer Research 68: 105–108

Spanos W J, Montague E D, Fletcher G H 1980 Late complications of radiation only for advanced breast cancer. International Journal for Radiation Oncology Biology and Physics 6: 1473–1476

Stephens F O, Crea P, Harker C J S, Roberts B A, Hambly C K 1980 Intra-arterial chemotherapy as basal treatment in advanced and fungating primary breast cancer. The Lancet II: 435–438

Stocks L H, Patterson F M S 1976 Inflammatory carcinoma of the breast. Surgery Gynecology and Obstetrics 143: 885–889

Stoker T A M 1974 The place of surgical excision in the management of locally advanced breast cancer. Cancer Treatment Reviews 1: 27–37

Stoll B A 1964 Rapid palliative irradiation of inoperable breast cancer. Clinical Radiology 15: 175–178

Strickland P 1973 The management of carcinoma of the breast by radical supervoltage radiation. British Journal of Surgery 60: 569–573

Whitehead R H, Thatcher J, Teasdale C, Roberts G P, Hughes L E 1976 T and B lymphocytes in breast cancer, stage relationship and abrogation of T-lymphocyte depression by enzyme treatment in vivo. The Lancet I: 330–333

Zucali R, Uslenghi C, Kenda R, Bonadonna G 1976 Natural history and survival of inoperable breast cancer treated with radiotherapy and radiotherapy followed by radical surgery. Cancer 37: 1422–1431

Index